PSYCHOTHERAPY IN AN AGE

OF NEUROSCIENCE

PSYCHOTHERAPY
IN AN AGE
OF NEUROSCIENCE

JOEL PARIS

Professor of Psychiatry, McGill University;
Research Associate, Department of Psychiatry,
Jewish General Hospital, Montreal, Canada

OXFORD
UNIVERSITY PRESS

Oxford University Press is a department of the University of Oxford. It furthers the University's objective of excellence in research, scholarship, and education by publishing worldwide. Oxford is a registered trade mark of Oxford University Press in the UK and certain other countries.

Published in the United States of America by Oxford University Press
198 Madison Avenue, New York, NY 10016, United States of America.

© Oxford University Press 2017

CIP data is on file at the Library of Congress
ISBN 978-0-19-060101-0

9 8 7 6 5 4 3 2 1

Printed by Webcom, Inc., Canada

*This book is dedicated to the teachers who encouraged
me to choose a career in psychiatry*

CONTENTS

ACKNOWLEDGMENT

Robert Biskin read an earlier version of this book and made many useful suggestions for improvement.

INTRODUCTION

In 1959, a chance encounter changed my life. I was an under-graduate studying psychology at the University of Michigan. One of the graduate students in the department, who also worked for the American Friends Service Committee, invited a group of students to spend a series of weekends at a nearby mental hospital. Ypsilanti State Hospital, now demolished, had at that time 4,000 patients, who were just beginning to be treated with effective drugs. Many had been there for years. I was fascinated by what I saw, and I decided that this was the problem to which I should devote my life.

I became a psychiatrist and have never been sorry about that decision. Mental illness remains mysterious, but mystery is what makes the field exciting. One of the things I loved best about psychiatry was that it was about both the mind and mental illness, straddling the boundary between normality and pathology.

Since my student days, psychiatry has changed—in some ways for the better but in some ways for the worse. One of the great mistakes of the past was to overprescribe psychotherapy and, when it did not help, to continue offering the same treatment, often for years. Now we have gone to the other extreme. Many psychiatrists spend little time listening to their patients. Our expertise is defined by the choice of drugs, which are now prescribed for almost everyone we see.

I have written this book out of a sense of loss and a feeling of hope. I was attracted to my profession by its breadth and humanism. My sense of loss comes from the fact that the field I loved has become narrow in scope, focusing almost exclusively on the biological factors in mental illness. There can be little doubt that modern psychiatry is much more scientific than it was in the past. We also know much more about neuroscience. But it is not obvious that this knowledge can be translated into practice or that our current treatments help more patients.

My feeling of hope comes from a belief that our current exclusive focus on biology is a phase that must pass. To deal with the complexity of the human mind and its disorders, psychiatry will need, in time, to return to a model of practice spanning the biological, psychological, and social aspects of mental illness.

Although this book focuses on my own profession, much of what I have to say is equally relevant to clinical psychology, to other mental health professions, and to primary care medicine. Psychologists have also been influenced by the current climate of opinion suggesting that all depressed patients should be on medications. Although physicians write most prescriptions, patients are often sent to us for consultation by psychologists asking for drugs to be added to the treatment regime. The result is, in a term famously applied to justifying a disastrous war, a "slam dunk."

I wrote a book some years ago about the state of contemporary psychiatry (Paris, 2008). However, the current volume differs in focusing on divisions within the field. I address two crucial questions. First, can neuroscience fully account for mental disorders, and to what extent can psychiatric treatment be based on this line of research? Second, in an age of neuroscience, does psychotherapy still have a role in psychiatry, and if so, how can it be integrated into practice?

I have no intention of trashing research in neuroscience, which, in the past few decades, has advanced by leaps and bounds. We knew little about the brain when I was a student. Now we are on the way to controlling the activity of individual neurons and to editing the genome itself.

The unanswered question is whether we know enough to apply this research to clinical practice. At this point, we do not. And there is another question that needs to be addressed. Even if we knew everything about the brain, would that knowledge be enough to explain how the mind works, or would we still need to study mental illness by measuring processes at a mental level? I am not a dualist, and I agree with neuroscientists that mind is what the brain does. But this book argues that thought, emotion, and behavior can never be fully explained by the activity of neurons, or their connections, and that these complex phenomena also need to be studied by considering the mind as a whole.

In the United States, the National Institute of Mental Health (NIMH), which directs research in psychiatry, has bet the farm on a project to explain all mental disorders as problems in neural connectivity (Insel et al., 2010). There can be no doubt that understanding brain circuitry will be of long-term benefit to psychiatry. But attempting to reduce mental illness to these mechanisms alone may be an illusory quest.

This line of research has thus far provided no benefit for patients who need better treatment now. While neuroscience has rapidly advanced, there has been little progress in applied sciences such as psychopharmacology. Moreover, by directing all research into a model based on a "connectome" (a system of neural connections), NIMH will largely exclude psychosocial research from funding. This decision follows the changing zeitgeist within psychiatry, marked by an almost religious belief in the primacy of neuroscience and a downgrading of everything psychological.

Neuroscience dominates psychiatry today—not because of its practical value but, rather, because of its glamor. The latest findings of research are trumpeted in the media. And since the media shape the way the public perceives science, patients today have come to expect medication from psychiatrists, and some demand an expertly mixed pharmacological cocktail.

Governments in North America and Europe are spending vast sums to support brain research. Neuroscientists have deservedly won several Nobel Prizes. But there is a large gap between basic and applied science. With the use of powerful new tools such as functional magnetic imaging, many leaders in psychiatry (e.g., Andreasen, 2001) have suggested that psychiatry is close to understanding how the brain works. This conclusion is very premature, and it is most likely wrong.

As a senior psychiatrist, trained in the late 1960s, I have lived long enough to see many trends come and go. But the most striking change in the field is that psychiatrists are no longer identified with the practice of psychotherapy. There has been a sharp decline in the use of psychological treatments among its practitioners (Marcus & Olfson, 2010;

Mojtabai & Olfson, 2008; Olfson & Marcus, 2010). Younger graduates learn about these methods but may not apply them. The culture of psychiatry works against psychotherapy. I have met psychiatrists who are openly disdainful of a "talking cure" and equate practicing "real" medicine with prescribing drugs. These clinicians restrict themselves to biological treatment and leave psychotherapy to psychologists and social workers.

Psychiatry now bases its legitimacy on its understanding of the brain and its ability to change the brain. It has therefore given up its traditional role as a humanistic discipline and has planted its flag on the territory of neuroscience. We now have an understanding of brain mechanisms that could only be dreamed of in the past. But this knowledge has not yielded progress in the treatment of mental disorders. We are often told that breakthroughs are just around the corner. But that is where they have remained.

The biological focus of modern psychiatry has a great advantage in the management of sicker patients. No one today would consider managing severe disorders such as schizophrenia or bipolar illness without a knowledge of psychopharmacology. Drug therapy remains the most important element of treatment for psychotic and severely depressed patients. But effective drugs for most of these conditions were developed approximately 50 years ago, long preceding the rise of neuroscience. Even today, we remain unsure how these agents work in the brain.

Psychiatrists also treat, or consult on, patients with less severe disorders. For this population, who suffer from what Goldberg and Goodyer (2005) call the "common mental disorders" (particularly anxiety and depression), a purely biological psychiatry has serious disadvantages.

Patients with common mental disorders may also benefit from pharmacotherapy, but the results are too often inconsistent. Psychotherapy is a robustly effective and evidence-based alternative for this population, supported by a very large body of research (Beck & Haigh, 2014; Lambert, 2013). Given this evidence base, managing patients with common mental disorders without psychological interventions is not good medicine. Many patients do well with no drugs at all, and the most comprehensive treatment for most common mental disorders is usually a combination of psychotherapy and pharmacotherapy. But there are important groups of conditions (addictions, eating disorders, and personality disorders) in which drugs play a minimal role and for which psychological interventions are the primary and most effective interventions.

This is why psychotherapy needs to remain in the armamentarium of psychiatrists in practice. I am not suggesting that we return to a past time when patients with less severe problems were seen weekly for years without obvious benefit. Instead, psychiatrists should provide brief and targeted therapies that research has shown to be effective. Moreover, some therapies can be provided without routinely applying a "split treatment," in which psychiatrists limit themselves to writing prescriptions while other professionals do the talking.

I do not view psychotherapy as a cure-all. It often fails. Many patients are unsuitable for talking therapy, and some therapists lack the skills to carry it out. But the track record of psychotherapy is more or less equivalent to that of antidepressants, which are widely prescribed despite their limitations. This book argues that keeping psychological therapy in the skill set of psychiatry leads to a more humanistic and effective practice.

I am fully aware that the need for psychotherapy will always be too great to be met by psychiatrists alone. I agree with those who believe that psychiatric expertise is too valuable a skill to be channeled into the care of patients whose problems can be effectively managed by other professionals. However, psychiatrists can work in teams, collaborating with clinical psychologists and social workers. They need to continue devoting themselves to the treatment of severely ill patients who absolutely require medical skills. But many of these patients, particularly those with personality disorders, substance use disorders, and eating disorders, need skilled psychotherapy.

I am a pragmatist. As an undergraduate and as a medical student, I observed the early days of antipsychotic treatment. As a resident, I was greatly impressed with the efficacy of electroconvulsive therapy, and I was the first physician at my hospital to administer lithium. However, by adopting a purely biological model, overprescribing medication to patients with common mental disorders, and failing to offer psychosocial treatments, psychiatrists are short-changing their patients. Psychiatrists have a responsibility to the mental health system that can be discharged by offering a wider range of treatments. That is the theme of this book.

PSYCHIATRY

Mindless or Brainless?

LEON EISENBERG (1922–2009) WAS A giant figure in 20th-century psychiatry, and he was often ahead of his time. In a much quoted article, Eisenberg (1986) noted that whereas the psychological theories that previously dominated psychiatry were "brainless" (lacking in grounding in neuroscience), the biological theories that replaced them were "mindless" (reducing all mental phenomena to cellular mechanisms). Eisenberg (2000) criticized the concept that mental disorders are *nothing but* brain disorders, which he viewed as narrowing the scope of psychiatry. This is also the point of view of this book.

Thirty years after Eisenberg's critique, biological psychiatry has become even more dominant. Some have applauded this shift as a return to our medical roots (Andreasen, 2001). Others have expressed concern that psychiatry has lost its humanistic core (Frances, 2013). Yet a return to psychiatry's identity as a medical specialty does not preclude humanism.

Research in neuroscience will eventually be of clinical benefit, but psychiatry is not based on neuroscience alone. Its scientific roots derive equally from biological and social sciences. That is what makes our specialty unique. Of particular concern, psychiatry has lost its connection to psychology, which should be one of its basic sciences. Research on abnormal psychology, or on psychotherapy, is only occasionally published in journals that psychiatrists read. Moreover, psychological constructs are sometimes viewed as fuzzy ideas that can be validated only by establishing correlations with biomarkers. The result has been that psychological theories are put on a back burner and practice focusing on psychosocial change has been marginalized.

In contemporary psychiatry, biological treatments are given a higher priority. That has happened because practitioners consider that their expertise lies in psychopharmacology and because psychotherapy is no longer part of their clinical culture. In a famous case from the 1980s, when medication was not offered to a hospitalized patient with severe depression, the failure to prescribe became grounds for litigation, which some experts found fully justified (Klerman, 1990). But no psychiatrist has ever been sued for failing to offer psychotherapy.

There have always been two kinds of psychiatry. After World War II, a book by a sociologist and a psychiatrist (Hollingshead & Redlich, 1958) described two types of practitioners. The "directive–organic" type wore a white coat and prescribed medication, whereas the "analytical–psychological" type wore a sport jacket and practiced psychotherapy. These distinctions never entirely disappeared. Mental health treatment split into two extreme positions, making the middle ground difficult to sustain.

Clinical practice among psychiatrists has come to focus exclusively on psychopharmacology. This is due to psychiatry's new identity as the clinical application of neuroscience

(Insel & Quirion, 2005). And although many practitioners report that they continue to provide psychotherapy (Mojtabai & Olfson, 2008), it is not always clear what they mean. (I cannot help but wonder if they are describing taking a few minutes to talk to patients whose prescription is being re-evaluated.) In any case, it is likely that only a minority offer evidence-based forms of psychotherapy. Methods such as cognitive–behavioral therapy require time and skill, and they are rarely integrated into psychiatric practice. Moreover, although physicians can refer patients to trained psychologists, they may fail to do so, preferring instead to pursue pharmacological treatment more aggressively.

PSYCHIATRY AND NEUROLOGY

Psychiatric theory and practice have moved from one extreme to another. History illuminates why. Like the rest of medicine, psychiatry began as a biologically oriented specialty (Shorter, 1997). Approximately 100 years ago, the hope was that, as had happened in internal medicine, diseases of obscure etiology and uncertain treatment would in time be explained by the discovery of anatomical or physiological biomarkers. But no one could find any correlates in the brain for mental illness. That was deeply discouraging. In the absence of effective treatment for severe disorders, therapeutic nihilism afflicted psychiatry.

Not all patients who came to psychiatrists in the past suffered from severe mental illness. A niche had long existed in medical practice for the treatment of "nervousness." These cases suffered from what we would now call common mental disorders, marked by mild to moderate anxiety and depression. In the 19th century, management of this population fell within the domain of neurology. Sigmund Freud, a neurologist by training, developed psychoanalysis to treat these patients.

Gradually, psychiatry split off from neurology. Although both specialties were concerned with brain disorders, neurology has always prided itself on its ability to find lesions that could be localized and that could account for symptoms. But no lesions or biomarkers are known to be consistently associated with mental disorders. Those that have such markers (e.g., dementia due to Alzheimer's disease) tend to be taken over by neurology or other branches of medicine.

Another factor in the split between psychiatry and neurology was that these specialties were rooted in different clinical settings (Scull, 2015). Psychiatrists were located in either mental hospitals or private offices; the move into general hospitals occurred later. One field was devoted to diseases of the brain associated with known physical changes, whereas the other was devoted to disorders of the mind (and brain) whose biological nature was unknown. It was also realized that whereas neurological diseases can be exclusively due to brain lesions, psychosocial factors play an important role in most mental disorders.

Today, practitioners take the division of labor between psychiatry and neurology for granted. In recent years, psychiatrists requiring board certification in psychiatry have no longer been required, as they once were, to take a separate examination in neurology. Yet some psychiatrists (Yudofsky & Hales, 2002), as well as some neurologists (Price, Adams, & Coyle, 2000), believe that the split was a mistake that perpetuated mind–brain dualism. They think that it is only a matter of time before the causes of severe mental illness will be localized in the brain.

The most influential voice supporting the reuniting of psychiatry and neurology has been that of Thomas Insel (1952–), Director of the National Institute of Mental Health (NIMH) from 2002 to 2015. In a widely quoted article published in *JAMA* (Insel & Quirion, 2005), he went on record as favoring making two specialties into one. Insel's view is that if mental disorders are brain disorders, there is no fundamental difference between psychiatry and neurology. The article by Insel and Quirion was also notable in defining psychiatry as an application of clinical neuroscience—as opposed to an integration of neuroscience and social science. The article does not even mention psychology.

Insel did not create this climate of opinion, but he reflects it. Given his many years of authority to direct the future of psychiatric research, Insel's views have been very influential. They were the seed for a neuroscience-based system of classifying mental disorders, the Research Domain Criteria (RDoC), currently being promoted by NIMH (discussed later).

In my view, reuniting psychiatry and neurology amounts to the abolition of psychiatry. As pointed out by Pies (2005), not all medical disciplines are located in a specific organ (immunology and oncology are examples). Moreover, psychiatry is fundamentally different in its understanding of illness from neurology. Once absorbed into a branch of medicine that has traditionally shown little interest in psychosocial factors affecting illness, all the unique aspects of the field will disappear (Zachar, 2000). In a phrase coined during the Vietnam War, those who favor this option think that to save psychiatry, it is first necessary to destroy it.

THE NEW BIOLOGICAL PSYCHIATRY

Psychiatry began as a biologically oriented discipline, but its failure to help most of its patients led to a turn toward psychological thinking. Then, in the second half of the 20th century, a second biological psychiatry appeared, based on the power of a new generation of drugs, reinforced by increased knowledge about the brain (Shorter, 1997).

The drugs came first. Yet after more than half a century has passed, we still do not know how these agents work in the brain. Yes, they affect neurotransmitters and their receptors. But no one has shown that neurochemistry accounts for their mechanism of action on the mind. As discussed in Chapter 2, there is much evidence *against* "monoamine hypotheses" as simple explanations for schizophrenia, mania, or depression.

Yet as long as drugs work, nobody need complain. The discovery of effective drugs in psychiatry was one of the greatest achievements in the history of medicine (Healy, 2002). But we should not fool ourselves into thinking that pharmacological mechanisms lead to an understanding of the causes of mental disorders or explain how drugs work. We should also keep in mind that the agents we use today are no more effective than those developed 60 years ago— they just have fewer side effects. That is a blessing, but newer drugs are not nearly as efficacious as pharmaceutical companies would like us to believe.

Neuroscience has grown in many ways during the past 40 years. The most potentially clinically relevant breakthrough is functional magnetic resonance imaging (fMRI). This technique measures brain activity by detecting changes associated with blood flow, allowing us to see the brain in action, at least to the extent that the rate of metabolism at various sites reflects mental activity. Even so, this tool, although powerful, only provides us with a broad sketch of brain function.

Neuroscience remains in its infancy. How could it be otherwise? The human brain is the most complex structure in the known universe. It contains nearly 100 billion neurons. The number of its interconnections has been estimated at 100 trillion. It also contains billions of glia whose functions are just beginning to be understood. The 1990s were called "the decade of the brain," but the complexity of the task probably requires a full century of research.

Because biological psychiatry is based on replicable scientific data, we can expect to *eventually* find answers to questions about how the brain works. However, experts keep promising breakthroughs that have not happened, and they may not happen within our lifetimes. The answers to our questions do not lie "just around the corner." Moreover, even if we knew everything about brain functioning, we would still need to study the mind at a mental level. Thought, behavior, and emotion are too complex to be reduced to neural mechanisms.

THE HARD PROBLEM, REDUCTIONISM, AND EMERGENCE

The relationship of mind and brain has long been a puzzle for scientists. Are mind and brain identical? Is it possible to reduce all mental activity to the activity of neurons and the connections between them?

Neuroscientists, psychiatrists, and philosophers have attempted to address these questions. David Chalmers (1996), an Australian philosopher and cognitive scientist, called the study of consciousness (reflecting the relationship between mind and brain) "the hard problem"—compared to the easier (albeit largely unsolved) questions facing neuroscience.

The hard problem could have several possible answers. One, held by many religions and some philosophers, is that mind and brain are entirely different. That would be an example of philosophical *dualism*. However, modern science firmly rejects dualism and can never accept the idea of a soul separate from the body. It adheres to *materialism*—the principle that all phenomena, including consciousness, are the result of material interactions.

A second answer to the hard problem could be that mind, consciousness, and thought are *epiphenomena* of brain processes that fully explain them. Following the scientific principle of *reductionism*, complex phenomena would be understood by reducing them to simpler components so that mind would be reduced and explained by brain functions (Gold, 2009). In this view, the best way to study mind would be through neuroscience, by understanding the chemistry and connectivity of the neurons that produce mental activity.

Reductionism is a basic principle in science. Atomic nuclei are made of quarks, chemical molecules are made of atoms, and living organisms are made of physical and chemical structures. In each case, understanding how components work has been the focus of research in physics, chemistry, and biology.

Reductionism has been one of the most successful of all scientific strategies. Examples include quantum theory in physics, Mendeleev's table in chemistry, and cellular mechanisms in biology. Reductionism has been equally successful in medicine. Prominent examples include heritable diseases that follow Mendelian genetics, as well as diseases with systemic effects that reflect the functional failure of specific organs or of cells within organs.

However, breaking down complex phenomena into simpler components faces the problem that there may be no point at which further reduction is possible. It is as if one had to open an endless series of Russian dolls. The physicist Arthur Eddington (1928) noted that the solidity of a table is in a certain sense an illusion, in that it is composed of atoms and mostly of empty space. But for practical purposes, it is legitimate to view a table as a table. In the same way, there are some questions about mind that cannot be answered by brain mechanisms alone. Thought, behavior, and emotions are emergent properties that can be studied in their own right.

Can reduction solve the hard problem? Some have thought so. Neuroscientists Paul and Patricia Churchland founded a field they call "neurophilosophy" (Churchland, 1986). Their version of reductionism goes far beyond the view that mind and body are identical. The Churchlands recommend eliminating psychology entirely as a discipline. They dismissively refer to its concepts as "folk psychology"—that is, purely intuitive ideas that must be reduced to the effects of variations in neural connectivity, which are more real. In this version of reductionism, mental phenomena are not worth studying because they can be eliminated by reduction to a neural level of analysis (Gold, 2009).The Churchlands' rejection of psychology may seem extreme. Yet it is not, as will be seen, very different from the ideas that dominate contemporary psychiatry.

Reductionism is the mainstream view of most neuroscientists—and of many psychiatrists. Philosophers actually describe multiple types of reductionism, depending on how strongly simpler components are thought to account for complex phenomena (Schwartz, Lilienfeld, Meca, & Sauvigne, 2016). The concept everyone would agree on is *constitutive reductionism*, which simply states that the mind is what the brain does. This would leave open the need for analysis on other levels and for the study of interactions between brain and environment. In contrast, *eliminative reductionism* suggests that all aspects of mental activity can be accounted for by study of the brain and that no other kind of science is needed.

There is a third possible answer to the hard problem, which is the answer that I favor. Mind is an *emergent* property of the brain's complexity. In other words, the concepts of mind and brain are not fully equivalent because they examine mental activity at different levels. The scientific study of nature has a kind of hierarchy: quarks, subatomic particles, atoms, molecules, cells, organisms, and societies. Each of these levels would be worth studying on its own, but none can be fully reduced to another. The same principle applies to the study of mind and brain. Just as one cannot fully explain chemistry by quantum physics, one cannot fully explain the mind by neural chemistry or connectivity.

The American philosopher Daniel Dennett (1996) coined the phrase "greedy reductionism" to criticize glib reductions of complex phenomena to simpler processes. Problems develop when scientists underestimate additional complexities that depend on interactions that cannot be accounted for by applying simpler levels of analysis.

The larger issue is that complex systems have characteristics that cannot be explained by reducing them to their components. These are their emergent properties (Kauffman, 1993). In other words, the whole is greater than the sum of its parts, and the whole cannot be reduced to its parts.

Biological systems have unique characteristics at different levels of organization (Deacon, 2011). Among the most important are order and self-regulation, which can arise spontaneously in complex systems (Kauffman, 1995). If it were not for the emergence of spontaneous order, it would be difficult to explain the evolution of the human brain.

Finally, reductionist models of mind and brain assume a one-way traffic pattern in which neurons create thoughts, emotions, and behavior. This view ignores the possibility that traffic can go the other way and that life experiences can change the brain. This process has been called *neuroplasticity*. This concept simply states that brain structure and function can change over time in response to changes in the environment. One well-supported concept, first developed by Hebb (1949), is that neurons that fire together, wire together. There is also good evidence for neurogenesis in some parts of the brain (Pascual-Leone, Amedi, Fregni, Merabet, 2005). A popular book by Doidge (2007) suggested that neuroplasticity could also be a model of how psychotherapy works.

All these complexities make neuroscience research on mental disorders unusually difficult. They provide a reason why it is unlikely that dramatic breakthroughs will take place in the near future. We need to understand what neuroscience can and cannot do. It can help illuminate how the mind works (Pinker, 1997), but we still need to measure mental processes to understand what the brain actually does (Burton, 2014).

Let us consider some analogous circumstances in the history of science. In the 1950s, biology became the most exciting area of scientific research. James Watson and Francis Crick announced their discovery of the structure of DNA in 1953. The genetic code was deciphered approximately a decade later, and mapping of the human genome was more or less completed by 2000. This was one of the greatest triumphs in the history of science.

The romance of molecular biology attracted many young people into the field. There was even a migration into biology of scientists from other disciplines. One was Francis Crick, originally trained in physics, who, as mentioned previously, became the co-discoverer of DNA and who was involved with unraveling the genetic code and spent the latter part of his career searching for the neural basis of consciousness (Crick, 1995). Not surprisingly for someone with his background, Crick was a strong reductionist who assumed that mental activities could be located in specific brain regions. He may have hoped to earn a second Nobel Prize by identifying the neural basis of consciousness. Unfortunately, Crick underestimated the complexity of the problem.

The power and glamor of genetics became so great that other forms of biology became a target for reductionist critics. In his autobiography, the entomologist Edward O. Wilson (1994) described what it was like being a biology professor at Harvard University when James Watson worked there. Colleagues called Watson "Caligula" because of his aggressive dismissal of any line of research in biology that was not molecular. (Although Wilson has studied chemical communication in ants, he is not a greedy reductionist.)

Reductionism in biological sciences was influenced by its previous success in physical sciences. Approximately

100 years ago, physics became an exciting discipline when it successfully showed how atomic theory accounted for many of the features of matter. Quantum theory allowed for even more precise predictions. The 20th-century physicist Ernest Rutherford has been quoted as stating, "All science is either physics or stamp collecting" (https://en.wikiquote.org/wiki/Ernest_Rutherford). To be fair, Rutherford was working at a time when much of biology was descriptive. Even so, it was surprising for a leading scientist to be so reductionist as to ignore one of the greatest ideas in the entire history of thought—Charles Darwin's theory of natural selection.

Natural phenomena depend on a system so complex that it cannot be reduced to a few simple components. Again, the key concept in understanding complex systems is emergence (Bedau & Humphreys, 2008)—that is, that systems have different characteristics at different levels of analysis. New characteristics are particularly likely to emerge when systems reach high levels of complexity. Thus, atoms are more than a collection of quarks and electrons, molecules are more than atoms, cells are more than molecules, and organisms are more than cells. Even if we knew how to describe all its connections, the brain would still be much more than the sum of its neurons.

Reductionism is most "greedy" when it attempts to reduce the social sciences to physical sciences. Yet if psychology were to be discarded in favor of biology, would we then take the next step and consider biology to be a branch of physics and chemistry? This leads to what philosophers call an *infinite regress*. Even the most hard-headed reductionist would not attempt to explain biology in terms of quarks or quantum mechanics.

The same constraint should apply to explaining the mind entirely in terms of biology (Schwartz et al., 2016). Of course, mental phenomena, whether normal or pathological, depend on processes in the human brain. The question is whether thoughts, emotions, and behaviors can be reduced to a neural level or whether complex systems have properties that can be fully accounted for by their components. No theory can be complete without understanding mental disorders at a mental level. Neuroscience is making a crucial contribution, but what could be most illuminating are interactive linkages between neural and psychosocial phenomena.

THE RDOC SYSTEM

One of the reasons why modern psychiatry has adopted a radically reductionist agenda derives from the limitations of models based on close observation of clinical phenomena. The *Diagnostic and Statistical Manual of Mental Disorders* (DSM) system (American Psychiatric Association, 2013) operationalized diagnostic criteria in psychiatry to identify patterns of psychopathology that could be reliably and directly observed but for which underlying biological mechanisms have not yet been identified. The hope was that biomarkers would eventually be found.

Yet despite decades of research within this framework, hardly any distinct biological mechanisms associated with discrete, categorically defined disorders were identified (Hyman, 2010). The DSM categories are too heterogeneous to be associated with endophenotypes or with specific etiological factors. Moreover, DSM has not even solved the problem of reliability, which remains low for most diagnoses, even for common categories such as major depressive disorder (Regier et al., 2013).

The National Institute of Mental Health developed RDoC as a way to organize research based on neuroscience, intended eventually to lead to a new diagnostic system (Cuthbert & Insel, 2013; Cuthbert & Kozak, 2013; Insel et al., 2010). The developers of the RDoC system reject the DSM approach and propose to replace it with a classification based on abnormal neural connections. They describe their aim as *translational* (Cuthbert & Insel, 2013)—that is, applying the findings of neuroscience to the understanding of the causes of mental disorders. Their strategy is to develop a matrix designed to describe the complex relationships between various levels and domains of psychopathology. With the aim of identifying fundamental components that span multiple disorders, RDoC has proposed seven "units of analysis": genes, molecules, cells, circuits, physiology, behavior, and self-reports. Based on these levels, the following five broad "domains/constructs" are suggested:

1. Negative valence systems (acute threat, potential threat, sustained threat, loss, and frustrative non-reward)
2. Positive valence systems (approach motivation, initial responsiveness to reward, sustained responsiveness to reward, reward learning, and habit)
3. Cognitive systems (attention, perception, working memory, declarative memory, language behavior, and cognitive control)
4. Systems for social processes (affiliation/attachment, social communication, perception/understanding of self, and perception/understanding of others)

5. Arousal/modulatory systems (arousal, biological rhythms, and sleep–wake)

These domains are derived from cognitive neuroscience models that have attempted to identify brain systems governing basic mental functions such as motivation, cognition, emotion, and behavior. However, few consistent relationships of this kind are known. Given the current state of research, requiring the use of the RDoC model for all future NIMH grant applications is very premature.

It is difficult to see how these five domains alone could account for the great variety of clinical symptoms associated with common mental disorders such as anxiety or depression, not to speak of severe mental disorders. Moreover, the key domains identified in RDoC all depend on abnormal neural connections or on interactions between environmental factors and neural structures. They make limited use of constructs that have been studied in psychology, developmental psychopathology, or social psychiatry.

By giving priority to neural circuitry (the "connectome"), RDoC proposes to account for symptoms affecting behavior, emotion, and cognition (Insel & Scolnick, 2006). Under Insel's leadership, NIMH invested $30 million in a "Human Connectome Project" (van Essen & Barch, 2015). The assumption is that the mind can be understood using a computational model of the brain (Friston, Stephan, Montague, & Dolan, 2014). (The newly appointed director of NIMH, Joshua Gordon, is associated with this line of research.) By defining psychopathology in this way, RDoC tends to institutionalize reductionism.

The RDoC system focuses on multiple levels of biological analysis (reflected in five of the seven specified levels), whereas psychological and social levels are represented sketchily and downplayed (Kirmayer & Gold, 2012). This bias ignores substantial areas of psychiatric research that examine the role of psychological and social factors in mental disorders (Paris & Kirmayer, 2016). Kirmayer and Crafa (2014) suggested that these limitations "are not accidental but stem from disciplinary commitments and interests that are at odds with the larger concerns of psychiatry" (p. 438). The model also ignores the science of complex systems with hierarchical structures (Kaufmann, 1995). Danish psychiatrist Josef Parnas (2014) described the RDoC system as "psychiatry without the psyche."

Yet it is possible to develop models that take both neuroscience and psychology into account. Mental disorders might be best understood as the result of interactions between brain structures and the social environment in which the mind develops (van Os, Lataster, Delespaul, Wichers, & Myin-Germeys, 2014). The neural reductionism of RDoC is an ambitious but ultimately invalid attempt to explain complex systems by simplifying causal pathways. These interactive processes are unlikely to be fully explained at the level of the genome or at that of neural connectivity (Melioni & Testa, 2014).

RDoC is very much in tune with the aim of psychiatry to emulate other medical specialties by focusing on the physiological and biochemical mechanisms that underlie disease. Yet even within the bounds of biological psychiatry, its view is much too narrow. One senior researcher (Carroll, 2015) argued for retaining the DSM approach, at least for now:

> Abandoning clinical diagnosis in research is ill-advised. The complex RDoC matrix bids fair to devolve into abstruse

metaphysical schematics, like the eccentrics and epicycles of 16th-century astronomy. A more productive path would be to promote iterative studies of potential biomarkers, using course of illness, family history, and response to treatment as convergent validators. (p. 1)

Moreover, despite advances in imaging technology, the mechanisms of complex mental functions remain largely inaccessible to neuroscience. To access the mind, we must still ask people what they are thinking and feeling (Burton, 2014). Although biological variables do shed important light on mental functioning, these measures lack meaning outside a psychological context. Yet RDoC has very little to say about psychology (Lilienfeld, 2014).

By seeing all psychopathology as *intrinsic,* RDoC makes a radical break with the biopsychosocial model and is more consistent with what Bentall (2010) ironically called the "bio-bio-bio" model of mental disorders. No one challenges the principle that all mental phenomena have neural correlates. However, this need not mean that psychological levels of analysis are irrelevant or unnecessary. The system does not consider extensive research on psychotherapy (Goldfried, 2015). It also excludes services research, which has helped define what clinicians require to manage difficult cases (Kane et al., 2016; Wunderink, Neboer, Wierma, Sytema, & Nienhuis, 2013).

Frances (2014) described RDoC as a useful initiative but one that is unlikely to provide short-term benefits. He accepts that neuroscience will eventually provide clinical benefits. However, Frances is critical of NIMH for ignoring the needs of patients who are poorly served by the current mental health system. He suggests, ironically, that because it is more interested in the brain than in mental health, NIMH should change its name.

Many psychologists, some of whom spend much of their professional lives validating measures of the mind, have been skeptical about RDoC (Lilienfeld, 2014). In a particularly cogent critique, Peterson (2015) noted that measures of mental phenomena of any kind are expected to have construct validity, discriminant validity, and predictive validity. But RDoC has little at this point but face validity, which is to say it looks more or less like what it proposes to measure. Finally, considering psychosocial factors in mental disorders only as epiphenomena of neural processes will prevent RDoC from answering the very questions it set out to explore.

The history of biological psychiatry has been marked by a pattern of overconfidence. Kraepelin (1919) expected the biological basis of psychosis to be found either during his lifetime or during the following generation. Almost 100 years later, we still have no answers to the most basic questions about mental illness. A prominent medical researcher, John Ioannidis (2015), stated the following about the current impasse in the understanding of psychopathology:

> I have great respect for etiologic and basic research, but I am afraid that there is substantial hype and such research may often not be as informative as it is expected to be. In the translational spectrum, the vast majority of funded and published research is basic, discovery T0 research, with a steep stepwise decline as we move to T1, T2, T3, and T4 research. . . . A key premise upon which the entire foundation of biomedical research enterprise has been based is the . . . claim that medical progress depends on biomedical research. . . . Human health has probably benefited more from nonmedical and non-basic-biomedical research-informed interventions than

it has from interventions that emerged from a pipeline that started with a basic biomedical, wet lab discovery. Hygiene, public health, computer science, engineering, transportation, and social constructs ... probably far outweigh in importance for health the best Nobel-caliber contributions of wet lab "basic" science. As we seek to curtail the burden of mental disease, perhaps we need less focus on studying the minutiae of extreme biological complexity and more on these other aspects that may make more of a difference. (pp. 241–242)

In other words, psychiatry should not expect neuroscience alone to answer all its questions but, rather, look for an integration of research from many different fields. Everyone can share in the enthusiasm about recent progress in neuroscience and cognitive science. However, the brain is too complex to give up its secrets easily. Again, this is not a project for a decade but, rather, for a century.

MENTAL DISORDERS AND BRAIN DISORDERS

Psychiatry has always been different from specialties such as internal medicine or surgery. It does not deal with diseases whose diagnosis can be confirmed by blood tests, imaging, or biopsies. Psychiatry concerns disorders of the mind—abnormalities in thought, emotion, and behavior that have not, despite great effort, been shown to have consistent biological markers.

The current "mantra" in psychiatry is that mental disorders are brain disorders (Insel et al., 2010). This is true in the sense that all mental phenomena are based on neural mechanisms. But it is only a half-truth. The other half of this story is that because mental disorders are related to emotions and behavior, they differ fundamentally from neurological disorders. In a meta-analysis, Crossley, Scott, Ellison-Wright, and Mechelli (2015) found that neurological disorders affect different brain circuits than those affected by mental disorders. The current mantra also begs the question as to whether mental disorders can be fully described by circuitry. Although a stroke can paralyze one side of the body, it may or may not have predictable or comparable effects on thought.

Whatever biological dysfunction underlies psychopathology, it will be mediated by the extraordinary complexity of the human mind. Moreover, biological mechanisms can only be understood in the context of specific environments. In a classic book on the scope of psychiatry, McHugh and Slavney (1998) argued that mental disorders require multiple, not single, models: the concept of disease, the concept of dimensions, the concept of behaviors, and the concept of life stories. This solution need not be seen as only provisional but, rather, as addressing the nature of an unusually complex discipline.

Nonetheless, influential voices favoring biology have dominated the debate. Francis Crick (1994) argued the case for reductionism in a challenging way: "You, your joys and ambitions, your personality, identity, and free will, are in fact no more than the behavior of a vast assembly of nerve cells and their associated molecules" (p. 3). With due respect to a great scientist, Crick's ideas about the mind were rather naive. (It is equally true that nerve cells and associated molecules can be seen as "no more than" the behavior of the atoms and subatomic particles that constitute them.) Crick was no doubt influenced by his previous discoveries, which replaced the vague idea of a gene with a specific molecule, DNA. But he failed to understand that good science is conducted using different perspectives and different levels of analyses, each of which can be valid.

Neuroscience has also been used to support the idea that free will is an illusion (Glannon, 2015). This conclusion seems to follow from the principle that mental phenomena can be entirely reduced to brain activity. Moreover, no specific place in the brain corresponds to our sense of a conscious self that directs our choices and our actions. Some have argued that neuroscience, by showing that brain activity changes prior to conscious awareness of a decision (Libet, Gleason, Wright, & Pearl, 1983), has disproved the existence of free will. This kind of determinism tends to support a purely biological psychiatry, in which patients become passive recipients of medication and their only role is to be compliant with prescriptions.

Psychiatry has traditionally taken a very different view. Without free will, much psychiatric treatment would be impossible. The practice of psychotherapy assumes that people can *decide* to change their lives. The recovery movement, particularly Alcoholics Anonymous, has adopted that point of view. The legal system would also collapse if it were generally believed that human behavior is nothing but the effects of brain activity. My own clinical team works with personality disordered patients, for whom one of the goals of therapy is to reduce victimization and increase agency. If we were strict reductionists, we would be forced to agree with our patients that they are victims of circumstance, and we would be unable to do this work.

In summary, neuroscience illuminates mental disorders but cannot explain them. It makes no more sense to reduce the mind to neurons than to explain neurons by quantum physics. With time, new paradigms could emerge that will allow us to know more than what is possible today. But even if that were to happen, mind and brain can never be understood outside a psychosocial context. This is because the brain is constantly changing under the impact of the environment. Even the size of the human brain is an adaptation to a complex social environment—a concept called the *social brain* hypothesis (Dunbar, 2014).

The American neurologist Robert Burton (2014), in a critique of the current overenthusiasm for neuroscience, notes that practitioners have no direct access to the mind but, rather, must rely on information about thoughts and emotions through questions and observations. It is wrong to assume that brain scans are somehow more "real" than what people have to say about inner states of mind or that fMRI results cannot be used to describe thought (Poldrack, 2006).

The idea that mental disorders are brain disorders also has an important political dimension. Family and consumer groups have adopted this idea to reduce stigma. It has been helpful to patients with severe illness, who should not be blamed for their symptoms. But the idea is less appropriate for patients with common mental disorders. Reducing depression and anxiety to brain abnormalities makes patients into victims, ignoring the ways in which people can change their life circumstances and their reactions to adversity. A purely biological view of depression and anxiety also encourages patients to be passive consumers of drugs rather than active agents in their own recovery.

Thus, the idea that mental disorders are brain disorders is at best a truism and at worst seriously misleading. It has become a dogma that creates as many problems as it solves. Psychiatrists, unlike most other physicians, can effectively treat some patients without drugs. Yet the idealization of neuroscience has led them to downplay psychological interventions that have as strong an evidence base as pharmacological agents.

The assumption is that once we understand the brain sufficiently, we will be able to treat mental disorders by modifying the activity and connection of neurons. However, the complexity of the brain makes this goal impractical. Moreover, reducing psychological symptoms to aberrant synapses fails to consider the emergent properties of the mind that cannot be explained at a neural level.

It is tempting to view mind as a fuzzy construct that needs to be reduced to simpler mechanisms. It is also tempting to diagnose patients, rightly or wrongly, with conditions that are known to be responsive to medication, such as major depression, bipolar disorder, or attention deficit hyperactivity disorder (Paris, 2015b). Currently, because psychiatrists define themselves as expert pharmacologists, diagnoses most likely to respond to psychotherapy, such as personality disorders, may not even be considered. The result is that many patients do not receive the best treatment.

CONSEQUENCES OF A BRAINLESS PSYCHIATRY

Brainless psychiatry, in which psychotherapy plays the major (or only) role in treatment planning, is rarely seen today, but it was very common when I entered resident training. Under the influence of psychoanalysis, this view was held with religious fervor. But it had serious clinical consequences in that patients who could benefit from medication were not necessarily offered the best options. As discussed previously, the case of a physician with melancholia who was not prescribed the antidepressants that later led to his recovery had a great impact on opinion in the field (Klerman, 1990). It also helped establish the principle that patients have a *right* to evidence-based treatment.

Even in the days of brainless psychiatry, it was common for patients in psychotherapy to receive some form of psychopharmacology, sometimes from a different physician. This use of "split treatments" has become more common now, in a time when psychologists do most of the therapy and when primary care physicians are comfortable prescribing antidepressants.

Psychiatric treatment, in any form, has to be accountable. Psychotherapy is a potentially powerful intervention, but it can sometimes fail or even do harm (Barlow, 2010). It should therefore be regulated as carefully as a drug. Clinicians should respond to failed therapy in the same way as they do when drugs fail—with a reassessment and a rethink.

Yet when I was in training, my teachers preferred to assume that when results are disappointing or partial, therapy has just not gone on long enough. This reminds me of the apocryphal saying, "The definition of insanity is doing the same thing over and over and expecting different results." In the absence of clear goals, defined outcomes, or accountability, psychotherapy can sometimes be disastrous. (This is why insurance companies and governments have been reluctant to insure it.) Psychotherapy failures are like treatment-resistant depressions in biological psychiatry, in that clinicians tend to expect too much from their interventions. These defects have long been clear for everyone to see, but there was a time when it was actually considered to be a virtue to be "brainless."

CONSEQUENCES OF A MINDLESS PSYCHIATRY

Mindless psychiatry leads to a different set of consequences. Because its practice excludes psychotherapy, it tends to resemble the way most other physicians see patients. A diagnosis is made, medication is prescribed, and further visits are used to monitor therapeutic effects and side effects or to add new drugs to the regime. These "med checks" focus entirely on symptoms, particularly when they correspond to criteria for a DSM diagnosis. Med checks last approximately 15 minutes, allowing psychiatrists to make much more money than by talking to patients for an hour. But in this time frame, little attention is given to exploring the life circumstances that often determine whether symptoms increase or decrease.

This is also the way that family physicians have learned to practice. My work as a consultant to primary care providers has brought these problems home to me. I frequently see patients who have been tried on three or four antidepressants, with an atypical psychotic added for "augmentation," all with minimal benefit. Often, no one has asked them how they are dealing with a recent loss, a job that has become more stressful, or a decline in physical health.

In a mindless psychiatry, patients are seen as problems in chemistry rather than in life. The proverbial (but scientifically invalid) concept of a "chemical imbalance" leads to treatment to restore the putative balance in neurotransmitter levels. This kind of practice fails to address the circumstances that make people unhappy. It is nothing but bad medicine.

2

THE LIMITS OF NEUROSCIENCE

THE EARLY DAYS

As an undergraduate student, I majored in psychology. Everything about the mind seemed fascinating. Psychology was a broad field, but because I was interested in the brain, I entered a stream in "physiological psychology'" (an ancestor of modern neuroscience). Looking back on those days, I am struck by the obscurity of the function of many brain regions. (My research supervisor worked on the hippocampus, which was still a mystery because its relationship to memory was then unknown.)

Nonetheless, the 1950s was a time of rapid growth for neuroscience research. There was much excitement about the role of the limbic system in emotion and behavior. One of my teachers, James Olds, was famous for having found a "pleasure center" in the rat brain (later found to be sites with many dopamine receptors). Another professor, Ralph Gerard, opened an Institute for Mental Health Research and went on to found the Society for Neuroscience. That organization grew rapidly, and it currently sponsors one of the largest of all scientific meetings (nearly 40,000 attendees in 2015). Gerard is sometimes remembered for a quip that nicely reflects biological reductionism in psychiatry: "Behind every twisted thought is a twisted molecule" (as quoted in Healy, 2002).

Early work in neuroscience had, however, raised serious questions about the importance of localization of behavior in the brain. A Harvard psychology professor, Karl Lashley, put forward principles he called "mass action" and "equipotentiality" (Lashley, 1950). In this view, most mental processes are not fully localized but are widely distributed in the brain. For all the discoveries that have been made about the functions of specific brain structures, Lashley's challenge has yet to be fully addressed. When we look at a functional magnetic resonance imaging (fMRI), what we see are differences between regions, making the more active one "light up." But this does not mean that mental activity is strictly localized. On the contrary, almost all important circuits are widely distributed in the brain.

Attempting to make sense of the brain's complexity, researchers have applied metaphors drawn from contemporary technology. Initially, the brain was thought of as a kind of telephone circuit. Later, it was viewed as a kind of computer. The computational theory of the mind, popular in cognitive science, builds on that idea (Friston, Stephan, Montague, & Dolan, 2014). Pinker (2002) viewed the brain as a set of modules packed together like a Swiss Army knife.

But none of these metaphors do justice to an organ of enormous complexity, with trillions of synapses. Nor are these ideas readily translated to a level of understanding that could inform clinical practice. As Hyman (2012) neatly stated,

> The best-recognized obstacles to effective clinical translation in psychiatry include the complexity of the brain and

the associated challenge of connecting levels of analysis from molecules to cells, synapses, circuits, and thence to higher cognition, emotion regulation, and executive function. (p. 2)

In fact, despite all the triumphs of neuroscience during the past few decades, *none* of them have led to more effective treatment for mental disorders.

WHAT DO WE KNOW NOW ABOUT NEUROSCIENCE?

I now take the reader on a very brief tour of neuroscience and its methods. I focus not on what has been accomplished but, rather, what remains unknown, and why this research has not yet led to any clinical applications.

Research on the brain has always been difficult—in addition to being complex, the organ is relatively inaccessible. Technology is often a driver of scientific advances. Approximately 60 years ago, we had few tools to study neuronal activity. Even the electroencephalogram was never very useful in psychiatry because recordings from the scalp do not measure changes in deeper brain structures. But we now have ways of looking at all areas of the brain and assessing their function.

Neuroanatomy

In contrast to other organs, brain biopsies are rarely conducted. Moreover, postmortem examination of the brain in patients with mental disorders has not generally yielded useful information. Even today, when slices can be frozen and stored in brain banks, significant anatomical findings have been rare.

Moreover, changes in neuroanatomy tend to be subtle. Einstein's brain was of normal size, and it took more than 50 years after his death to find differences in the thickness of a few cortical areas (Men et al., 2014). And even then, this finding hardly explains why Einstein was a genius because there is little evidence (outside of intellectual deficiency) that brain size and structure have a strong correlation with intelligence. One can use imaging methods to conduct volumetric studies of the size of brain regions, but this approach has also been of limited value for the practice of psychiatry (Hyman, 2012).

Neurochemistry

Neurochemistry was one of the first areas of dramatic progress in understanding how the brain works. Until Nobel Prize-winning research in the 1960s by Julius Axelrod (Coyle, 2005), it was not known that catecholamines, whose receptors are the target of many psychiatric drugs, were involved in synaptic transmission. The discovery that glutamine and gamma-aminobutyric acid (GABA) account for 99% of transmission in all brain synapses is an even more recent discovery (Coyle, 2006). However, none of these discoveries came anywhere near to accounting for the causes of mental disorders or the mechanisms of treatment for these illnesses. In fact, there is little consistent evidence that specific neurotransmitters are abnormal in schizophrenia, depression, or any other major disorder.

Several promising leads have run cold (Hyman, 2014b). One is the theory that decreased serotonin activity causes depression; another is the hypothesis that changes in dopamine receptors are related to schizophrenia (Moncrieff, 2009). These ideas were developed by working backwards from the effects of drugs that block transmitter receptors. But research has found no evidence that the mechanisms of action of antipsychotics, antidepressants, or lithium are specifically related to these systems. To consider one example, specific serotonin reuptake inhibitors (SSRIs) raise mood, but so do drugs that augment the reuptake of serotonin (De Simoni, DeLuigi, Clavenna, & Manfridi, 1992). Moreover, antidepressants that inhibit the reuptake of both serotonin and norepinephrine are no more effective than those with a single action (Cipriani et al., 2009).

Recent research has also explored the important role of neuropeptides such as oxytocin and vasopressin (Panksepp & Harro, 2004). These molecules play a key role in emotion, but no clinical application has yet emerged from this line of investigation.

Although theories of psychopathology based on "chemical imbalances" of neurotransmitters have failed or been proved wrong, the simplicity retains a hold on physicians and patients. Psychiatrists who attend educational events sponsored by the pharmaceutical industry will be familiar with slides that expert speakers like to present at these conferences. They show the synapse in detail, with bright colors used to underline the putative mechanisms of drug action. At best, these diagrams are suggestive. At worst, they are fictional.

Theories about drug action in psychiatry are not used in the same way as in medicine, in which physicians conduct blood tests to monitor the effects of treatment. Psychiatrists can measure the level of drugs in the body but cannot evaluate how they are working in the brain. Most of the information we obtain about the outcome of treatment comes from low-tech measurements, such as clinician interviews and patient self-reports.

Neuroimaging

The most striking advances in neuroscience in recent years have come from neuroimaging. The introduction of brain scans is a perfect example of how technology drives research. Earlier research used computerized axial tomography (CAT scans); magnetic resonance imaging (MRI), which can measure the relative size of brain regions; as well as positron emission tomography (PET), which can identify the site of action of neurotransmitters. But with fMRI, which measures blood flow in specific regions, we can, at least indirectly, observe brain activity.

These techniques were immediately expected to play an important role in clinical psychiatry. When I worked under a Dean of Medicine whose specialty was immunology, he told me that future psychiatrists would carry out "bedside fMRI" to guide their choice of treatment. Twenty years later, this application to clinical practice remains out of reach. One reason is that there are limitations on what imaging can tell us about the brain. First, the method does not, as often claimed, show brain areas "lighting up." The data indicate only that metabolism is higher in some areas compared to other areas. These are statistical relationships that do not rule out Lashley's "mass action." Moreover, fMRI pictures mislead us with bright visuals, making use of artificial colors to highlight differences between regions. Data interpretation can often be difficult, with localization often unclear; it can even be difficult to differentiate excitation from inhibition (Logothetis, 2008).

Raz (2012), a researcher with experience in imaging research, described the problem as follows:

> fMRI studies frequently produce billions of data points—most of them sheer noise—wherein one can find coincidental patterns. Whirl those tea leaves around often enough and recognizable impressions will appear at the bottom of your cup. In addition, many fMRI studies dip into the same data twice: first to pick out which parts of the brain are responding; and second to measure the response strength. This practice is statistically problematic and results in findings that appear stronger than they actually are. (p. 268)

Moreover, samples in research studies tend to be very small (due to the cost of the procedure), and they may not be representative of clinical populations. Finally, as in all research, one should be on the lookout for publication bias—it is much more difficult to publish negative than positive findings (Dickersin, 1990).

Jerome Kagan, a senior developmental psychologist, has been a thoughtful skeptic about research that purports to localize thought in one or another brain region. Although there is little doubt about the overall function of the prefrontal cortex, Kagan (2006) concluded, "A critical review of 275 studies that used PET or fMRI revealed that several brain regions are engaged by most cognitive challenges. ... The prefrontal cortex should be regarded as a general computational resource" (p. 234).

fMRI is a powerful tool that may be further developed in the future to provide more precise data. But its current limitations need to be more widely understood (Satel & Lilienfeld,

2013). Perhaps the brilliant (but artificial) colors of these scans mislead us into believing that we are actually seeing "the brain in action." Imaging provides important clues to cognition, but it does not mirror thought (Poldrack, 2006).

Molecular Genetics

In 2000, scientists learned how to read the entire human genome, and they have been hard at work ever since to decode it. Hopes were high for a research breakthrough that would lead to better treatment for physical and mental illnesses. This enthusiasm failed to recognize certain limitations. One is the difference between simple Mendelian inheritance and the complex heritability associated with chronic diseases. Most diseases are correlated with a large number of small effects associated with a surprisingly large number of genes (Hyman, 2014a). Another is the fact that most genes do not code for proteins but, rather, are involved on a larger scale in the organization of genome functions.

With the development of gene therapy, it has been suggested that diseases could be either prevented or cured by changing the genetic code (Sapolsky, 2003). Although such advances are technically possible, phenotypes reflect environmental influences that are either not recorded in genotypes or can change gene expression. We are often told that we are near to achieving such goals, but again, breakthroughs always remain just around the corner.

The contribution of molecular genetics to psychiatry has thus far been minimal. Linkage and association studies, probably because they were searching for needles in haystacks, have been disappointing. Even using the more powerful technique of genome-wide association studies (GWAS), the most consistent finding has been that single genes, or groups of genes, do not account for a large percentage of the risk for any major mental disorder (Hyman, 2014a). Instead, genetic risk reflects interactions between large numbers of different genes, many of which are common variants and each of which accounts for only a small proportion of the variance. For example, a large-scale study of schizophrenic patients that was published in *Nature* (Schizophrenia Working Group of the Psychiatric Genetics Consortium, 2014; see also McClelland et al., 2007) found 108 genes potentially associated with the disorder, and none had more than a small effect. This principle seems to apply to all the complex features of the human brain.

Another reason why molecular genetics has been disappointing as a basis for practice is that although genes make pathology more likely, they do not predictably determine clinical outcomes. The complexity is further explained by the fact that changes in the genome can be turned on and off by molecular switches that are responsive to the environment (Meaney & Szyf, 2005). This *epigenetic* system, which is a feedback loop for gene–environment interaction, is just beginning to be understood (McGowan & Roth, 2015).

Some disorders are more heritable than others. Common mental disorders such as depression and anxiety have a genetic component, accounting for approximately half the variance (Kendler & Prescott, 2006). But that leaves another half of the variance that measures responses to environmental circumstances.

In recent years, it has been claimed that mapping the genome could allow psychiatrists to identify loci of change or polymorphisms that might constitute the genetic causes of mental illness (Cannon & Keller, 2006). It is also possible that the recent discovery of "gene editing" (Lundgren, Charpentier, & Fineran, 2015) could be applied to conditions with a Mendelian inheritance. Others have proposed that we are entering an era of "personalized medicine" in which, as has already happened for cancer patients, treatment can be adapted to individual genomes and their associated biomarkers (Cuthbert & Insel, 2013). However, thus far, these expectations have also met with disappointment. One reason is that biological risk may derive from many different pathways. Moreover, many genetic variations contribute risk to all kinds of mental health problems and not just to one disorder (Rutter, 2006). Finally, these theories fail to take environmental factors in disease into account.

In developmental psychopathology, the complex relationships between risks and outcomes have been called *equifinality* and *multifinality* (Ciccheti & Rogosch, 1996). In other words, different risks can lead to the same outcome, and the same risk factors can lead to different outcomes. In this light, it should not be surprising that the mapping of the human genome will not find simple correspondences between genes and complex (behavioral) phenotypes but, rather, shows that the genome itself is a complex dynamical system that responds in complex ways to developmental histories. We are just beginning to understand that genes rarely act alone but, rather, work together in a kind of "society" (Yanai & Lercher, 2016).

One can criticize biological psychiatry for trying to reduce mental disorders to variables measurable by neuroscience. Yet in the past, an equally absurd form of reductionism afflicted psychiatry—the idea that mental disorders are entirely due to adverse life experiences. An excessive focus on environmental factors in development has also characterized much of social science, which has tended to view the concept of heritability as overly pessimistic or even dangerous (Pinker, 2002). Both forms of reductionism are dubious.

Behavioral Genetics

Behavioral genetics is *not* a neuroscience method. Instead, it uses statistical data to quantitatively estimate the heritability of disorders and their underlying traits (Jang, 2005; Plomin, DeFries, Knopik, & Neiderhiser, 2013). Thus, although behavioral genetics does not concern itself with biological mechanisms, it has told us more about the heritability of mental disorders than has molecular genetics.

Behavioral genetics usually obtains its data by measuring differences between concordance for a disorder (or a trait) in monozygotic and dizygotic twins. The larger the difference between monozygotes and dizygotes, the higher will be the heritability. But because these estimates apply to populations, and not to individuals, heritability is not necessarily the same in all individuals.

Even so, behavioral genetics provides a "ballpark" overview of the relative contributions of genes and environment to the causes of psychopathology. It shows that approximately half the variance in most mental disorders is determined by heritable factors. Disorders that are more heritable (e.g., autism with 90% of the variance, and bipolar disorder and schizophrenia with 80%) contrast with those that are less heritable (e.g., major depression with 35–40%) (Burmeister, McInns, & Zollner, 2008).

Because half the variance of common mental disorders is *not* heritable, behavioral genetics also has something important to tell us about environmental factors in etiology.

First, contrary to classical psychological theories, the portion of the variance that derives from nonheritable factors is not "shared" (i.e., related to growing up in a particular family) but, rather, "unshared" (i.e., related to unique life experiences). Second, common mental disorders are much less heritable than are severe mental disorders. But *all* disorders, even the most severe, have a clinically relevant degree of influence from the environment.

THE BOUNDARIES OF OUR KNOWLEDGE

None of the methods for assessing biological factors in mental disorders have accounted for their etiology. At this point, it seems safe to say that breakthroughs, if any, are unlikely for decades to come. When the problem is this complex, researchers should not make promises they cannot keep.

Yet psychiatrists, and their patients, have been given the impression that neuroscience will answer their questions about illness and that it already explains how drugs for mental illness work. Although such discoveries could eventually emerge, at this point we just do not understand the mechanisms. Psychiatrists must accept that their biological treatments, even those that are most effective, are almost entirely empirical. Our drugs often work, and they often help patients, even if we do not know how.

Moreover, there is no reason to make sharp distinctions between nature and nurture. The best explanations of normal and abnormal behavior, emotion, and thought lie in models that take both into account (Paris, 1999). As Chapter 4 will show, interactions between genes and environment are the key to explaining why biological vulnerability does not necessarily lead to disorders and also why adverse life experiences can affect different people very differently (Kendler & Prescott, 2006; Rutter, 2000). Genes do not produce mental disorders, but they are an important part of the puzzle. The problem thus far in research has been studying genes and biomarkers without examining their interactions with the environment.

Some developments in neuroscience have sought to take these complexities into account. But they are still limited by adherence to a reductionist agenda. Thus, cognitive neuroscience (Gazzinaga, Ivry, & Mangun, 2002) and social neuroscience (Cacioppo, Cacioppo, Dulawa, & Palmer, 2014) have emerged as useful ways of accounting for thought and behavior on a basis of brain activity. However, these models tend to favor neural over mental processes and do not seriously consider that psychological and social mechanisms also shape the brain.

Kirmayer and Crafa (2014) have recommended a different approach. They argue that neuroscience cannot be a mature science without taking into account the evolution of a "social brain" (Dunbar, 2014). In this perspective, many of the most important functions of the human brain, and the reason for its large size, concern the management of complex interpersonal interactions. For example, reading other people's minds involves much more than the currently fashionable (but heavily hyped) concept of mirror neurons (Hickok, 2014). Moreover, it may not be valid to separate neural and social mechanisms or to define one in terms of the other. It is also not valid to treat patients for brain dysfunctions when their real problems lie in the interpersonal world they inhabit. Moreover, psychological and social events do not arise de novo from neural connections but, rather, actively shape the activity and structure of the brain.

This is the Achilles' heel of an overly ambitious neuroscience. It wants to explain as much as possible about human nature from the structure of the brain. With time, much more will certainly be known about how neural systems work.

Like everyone else, I applaud the triumphs of neuroscience. We are now moving into an era marked by further advances, such as gene editing (Lundgren et al., 2005) and controlling neurons with light beams (Deisseroth, 2011). Yet we are very far from applying these discoveries to clinical practice. Moreover, outside of a psychosocial context, neuroscience has little meaning. As Chapter 3 will show, reductionism of the mind to neurochemistry can also be a recipe for failed treatment.

3

PRESCRIBING

AND OVERPRESCRIBING

NEUROSCIENCE AND PSYCHOPHARMACOLOGY

The development of effective psychopharmacology was a heroic chapter in the history of medical science (Healy, 2002). Fifty to 60 years ago, patients benefited from a rapid development of efficacious pharmacological treatments for most severe mental disorders. This was a wonderful time to be in training to become a psychiatrist.

Antipsychotics appeared in the 1950s, followed by antidepressants, and by 1970, lithium became available. All of these medications were discovered by serendipity. Antipsychotics began as sedatives for anesthesia, antidepressants were first developed as antipsychotics, and lithium was originally a treatment for gout. To this day, our knowledge of how any of these drugs work in the brain is sparse and speculative—not surprising, given that neuroscience is still in its early days.

However, because psychiatric drugs usually (and sometimes dramatically) worked, they became the basis of a "psychopharmacological revolution." Patients who once might have spent years in hospital could now be discharged in weeks or, sometimes, a few days. Moreover, drug therapy could often be conducted in outpatient settings, avoiding hospitalization entirely. Traditional mental hospitals emptied out or closed down.

It was natural to expect more miracles to be on the way. However, progress during the past 40 years has been disappointingly slow. Most of the agents in current use are variants of older drugs, albeit with less problematic side effects.

For example, when atypical antipsychotics were introduced in the 1980s, psychiatrists were relieved that they did not carry a high risk for irreversible side effects, particularly movement disorders such as tardive dyskinesia that were associated with typical antipsychotics. Yet, despite initial claims, the newer drugs are no more effective for psychosis than the older drugs. Impressive data from the large-scale CATIE study (Lieberman et al., 2005), which compared the efficacy of typical versus atypical antipsychotics in schizophrenia, found no difference in outcome. Similar results emerged from a British study (Lewis & Lieberman, 2008). Although many psychiatrists were shocked that efficacy was the same (which is not what pharmaceutical representatives had been saying), practice did not change. Another reason for continued use of atypicals is that tardive dyskinesia is more worrisome than weight gain and metabolic syndrome.

The only atypical drug used today that has a special role in difficult cases is clozapine (Wahlbeck, Cheine, & Essali, 2000). Introduced in 1971, clozapine had been withdrawn in 1975 because of the danger of agranulocytosis, but it was brought back 10 years later because of its unique efficacy in schizophrenia.

Much the same can be said about the replacement of tricyclic antidepressants by specific serotonin reuptake inhibitors

(SSRIs), as well as serotonin–noradrenaline reuptake inhibitors (SNRIs). The use of these newer drugs meant that we need not worry so much about anticholinergic side effects or whether a patient could die by overdosing on a week's supply. But this did not make the newer drugs more effective. MacGillivray, Arroll, Hatcher, and Ogston (2003) compared the efficacy of tricyclic antidepressants and SSRIs and found minimal differences. There may be a minor advantage for tricyclics in severe depression (Anderson, 2000).

The story for the treatment of bipolar disorder is different. After half a century, lithium is still the first choice for bipolar patients (Geddes, Burgess, Hawton, Jamison, & Goodwin, 2004), and it may also help prevent suicide in this clinical population (Cipriani, Pretty, Hawton, & Geddes, 2005). Recently, it has become common to replace lithium with less toxic anticonvulsant mood stabilizers. But these agents are less effective than lithium, the older and cheaper alternative.

In short, if we had only the drugs that were available in the 1970s, we would still be able to treat most severely ill patients effectively. Newer drugs in psychiatry may be tolerated better but are not more effective.

THE PROBLEM OF OVERPRESCRIPTION

The lack of evidence for the superiority of new medications has not prevented the pharmaceutical industry from investing in them and actively promoting their use. For example, there are now a large number of SSRI antidepressants, as well as serotonin and several SNRIs, on the market. Yet comparative trials have found little or no evidence that any one of these agents is superior to any other (Cipriani et al., 2009; Gartlehner et al., 2008).

Antidepressants, prescribed for even the mildest depression, have been lucrative for industry. Given the high prevalence of major depression, and a tendency to longer term use of antidepressants, this is a very large market. (Industry has been reluctant to develop new antibiotics, which are badly needed, because they are taken for only a short time.) Moreover, the efforts of Big Pharma to encourage the use of antidepressants have largely been successful. But in the absence of real progress, the drive to promote "me-too" drugs has slowed in recent years, and industry has tended to invest in other areas of medicine.

Unfortunately, physicians tend to prescribe the most recent drugs at the expense of tried and true older ones. As a consultant, I am amazed by how many patients seen in primary care are prescribed the latest and most expensive agents. This is largely because drug representatives convince physicians that new agents are better. They also offer free samples to improve marketing. And when drugs go generic, their rate of prescription declines almost immediately (Avorn, 2004).

Between 11% and 13% of the population is currently on antidepressants (Kantor, Rehm, Haas, Chan, & Giovannucci, 2015; Pratt, Brody, & Gu, 2011), mostly for mood and anxiety disorders. (The majority of these prescriptions are not written by psychiatrists but, rather, by primary care physicians.) There are several reasons for the widespread use of antidepressant drugs. First, the bar for diagnosing major depression in the fifth edition of the *Diagnostic and Statistical Manual of Mental Disorders* (DSM-5; American Psychiatric Association, 2013) is low (five of nine symptoms for only 2 weeks). Thus, antidepressants may be prescribed for patients with mild symptoms who might be better described as unhappy with their lives. Second, antidepressants are heavily advertised, both to physicians and to potential patients. Third, antidepressants have strong placebo effects, which have increased throughout the years (Kirsch, 2014), probably due to marketing. Fourth, once patients are on these drugs, physicians and patients are reluctant to stop them for fear of symptomatic recurrence, so many stay on them for years. Moreover, as discussed later, it is common for patients who do not respond to antidepressants to be treated with complex polypharmacy regimes (Kingsbury, Yi, & Simpson, 2001). The outcome is that patients with depression end up receiving medications they may or may not need. Let us consider the strength of the evidence for their efficacy.

ARE ANTIDEPRESSANTS CONSISTENTLY EFFECTIVE?

Antidepressants are the mostly widely used psychiatric drugs in medicine, and they are among the most frequently prescribed medications of any kind. SSRIs, SNRIs, and tricyclics can all be helpful for depression (Moncrieff, Wessely, & Hardy, 2004; National Institute for Care Excellence, 2009), and they are also used for anxiety disorders, obsessive–compulsive disorder, and a variety of other conditions.

The key question is whether these agents work as well in mild to moderate depression as they do in severe depression. The best research, including meta-analyses, shows they have only a slim advantage over placebo in such cases and that initial severity is the best predictor of response (Fournier et al., 2010; Kirsch et al., 2008). In other words, the sicker the patient, the better these drugs work.

Some of the confusion about the effectiveness of these agents arises from the fact that patients with milder depressions tend to have strong placebo responses, whereas those with severe depressions show hardly any placebo response. Moreover, as patients and physicians have come to believe that antidepressants are the best answer to depressed mood, these responses have increased (Kirsch, 2014). The problem is that placebo effects, although initially impressive, rarely last for long.

The crucial point is that the efficacy of antidepressants for non-melancholic depression is not as high as many believe. This became more obvious once researchers obtained access to failed trials sponsored by industry that had never been published, largely due to unsatisfactory results (Fournier et al., 2010; Kirsch et al., 2008). At best, only 50% of depressed patients achieve full remission from pharmacological treatment (as opposed to a reduction in symptoms that is statistically, but not clinically, significant).

Physicians are prescribing these agents with unjustified confidence. Patients are given the impression that antidepressants yield predictable results for depressive symptoms. But while high expectations may increase short-term response, they by no means guarantee long-term improvement. We should be telling patients the truth: Medication works approximately half the time, and one can only know whether a drug will work by trying it. (Even then, it is impossible to know if one is observing a true therapeutic response or a strong placebo response.)

We would not know that the efficacy of antidepressants is less than believed if researchers had not dug more deeply into the data. Initial trials funded by industry offered misleadingly positive conclusions, but replications are rare. Moreover, some published reports are misleading. For example, a well-known trial of paroxetine in adolescents (Keller et al., 2001) was later shown to have failed to yield *any* effect when the data were carefully reanalyzed (LeNoury et al., 2015). The meta-analyses of Kirsch et al. (2008) and Fournier et al. (2010), indicating that most agents are only slightly better than placebo for mild to moderate depression, were based on a re-examination of unpublished data.

Thus, it is difficult to interpret clinical trials, and placebo effects make it even more difficult to establish causality in practice. Both physicians and patients tend to attribute changes, whether positive or negative, to drug prescriptions. (Our minds are designed to find patterns, whether they are or are not causally valid.) Often, a patient gets better and we attribute the improvement to a change of medication. But it may equally be explained by the hope aroused by the latest prescription and the patient's perception that the physician is "doing something." Improvement may also be due to a change in life circumstances or to naturalistic remission (particularly common in milder depressions).

When patients do not respond to medication (which happens in approximately half of cases), this does not prove that a depression is "treatment resistant." This term is misleading because it considers depression to be a biological phenomenon without considering its context. An alternative explanation is that drug treatment has simply had no effect on the stressors driving lowered mood. In other words, the pressure to treat all types of depressed mood with aggressive pharmacotherapy ignores the option of psychological investigation or psychotherapy. Instead, physicians tend to deal with treatment resistance by either changing drugs or adding new ones.

We usually speak of *treatment-resistant depression* (TRD) when antidepressants fail. But what we are actually seeing is resistance to psychopharmacology—not to all forms of treatment. The concept of TRD is based on the doubtful assumption that major depression is a diagnosis as real as pneumonia. (In that case, physicians correctly speak of antibiotic resistance.) Actually, major depression describes a heterogeneous group of patients, ranging from those who require hospitalization to people who are slow to recover from a life stressor (Paris, 2015b). It should therefore not be surprising that some patients on antidepressant drugs do better than others.

MISADVENTURES WITH AUGMENTATION AND SWITCHING

One of the problems in any field of medicine (or clinical psychology) is what to do when treatments do not work. Perhaps the diagnosis was wrong. Or patients may have comorbidities that were not targeted. There is good evidence, for example, that antidepressants are not very useful for patients who also meet criteria for personality disorders (Newton-Howes, Tyrer, & Johnson, 2006).

The larger error lies in considering DSM diagnoses as specific entities requiring specific treatment with drugs. The DSM manual is little but a convenient way of communicating about psychopath1ology in patients (Paris, 2015a). Severe illnesses resemble medical illnesses, but most diagnoses are syndromes, without specific etiologies or a specific course. Depression blends around the edges into unhappiness. It is only because we have used this diagnostic category for decades that we fall into the habit of treating it as a medical disease that always requires drug treatment.

A related error is to prescribe drugs for a "comorbid" depression found in conditions that do not respond well to pharmacological therapy. This assumes one can slice up symptoms into manageable bites, each of which has a unique pharmacological remedy.

Meta-analyses of antidepressant efficacy in major depression summarize the results of clinical trials. But drug effects are not always generalizable from randomized controlled trials (RCTs). The problem is that the patients who enter these trials are highly selected. Zimmerman, Mattia, and Posternak (2002) reported that only a minority of cases seen in clinics would meet research criteria for these trials, given that RCTs usually have exclusions for suicidality, substance abuse, or anxiety disorders.

One way to address this problem is to conduct *effectiveness* trials—naturalistic follow-up of unselected patients receiving well-defined treatment. The disadvantage of this method is the absence of a control group, making it impossible to determine whether remission would have occurred naturalistically (i.e., in the absence of treatment). If many cases of major depression remit spontaneously over time, the success of strategies to deal with treatment resistance will be clouded by the rate of spontaneous recovery. In a review, Khan and Brown (2015) noted, "The effect size of current antidepressant trials that include patients with major depressive episode is approximately 0.30 (modest), and this fact needs to be heeded for future antidepressant trials" (p. 299).

The Sequenced Treatment Alternatives to Relieve Depression (STAR*D) study was an effectiveness study designed to assess the effects of antidepressants in a real-world clinical sample of more than 4,000 patients. In a summary paper, Rush (2007) reported that only approximately 40% responded to a first course of antidepressant therapy. Although 70% of patients in the sample eventually remitted, it was not clear how many would have done so with no treatment at all. This rate does not correspond to remission rates in most clinical trials, which are approximately 50% (Kirsch, 2014). But the difference could be explained by the length of an effectiveness study, in which further improvement can be due to naturalistic remission. This research method (effectiveness rather than efficacy) could not distinguish gradual improvements that may or may not be related to drug therapy.

Overall, the results of STAR*D were discouraging for those who believe in prescribing drugs for every depressive episode. However, Rush (2007), who was one of the investigators, had a different spin on the data. He recommended that clinicians should not give up when drugs initially fail to produce results but, instead, try other agents, as well as augmenting drugs. This persistent approach has become standard practice. However, STAR*D showed that some patients continue to be "treatment resistant." Although STAR*D did examine a small group that was referred to cognitive-behavioral therapy (CBT), augmentation with psychotherapy was a very small part of the research design.

There could be other problems with the STAR*D data. In a critique, Pigott, Leventhal, Alter, and Boren (2010) noted difficulties in the study methods, including a failure to report a 10% drop-out rate after assessment and initial treatment, as well as counting patients who later relapsed as remitted. Correcting for these errors, Pigott et al. recalculated the overall remission rate as only 38%. That is closer to the response rate in meta-analyses comparing antidepressants to placebo (Kirsch et al., 2008). Moreover, as noted by Plakun (2015), patients in this effectiveness study had comorbidities that are usually excluded from clinical trials, which might explain their lower rates of improvement (39%) or remission (25%) in the short term.

The idea of TRD (Papakostas & Fava, 2010) is derived from the artificial setting of clinical trials with selected patients. However, because severe depression responds better than mild to moderate depression to antidepressants, one might get entirely different results in hospitalized patients.

Current practice uses several strategies to deal with TRD. One is *switching*—that is, changing to another antidepressant when the first choice fails. Although patients can have idiosyncratic responses to drugs, meta-analyses of head-to-head comparisons of antidepressants have found almost no difference in efficacy (Cipriani et al., 2009). When STAR*D examined the effects of switching, some patients who failed to respond to one antidepressant did better on another one. However, it was not worth trying more than one switch because doing so had diminishing returns (Rush, 2007). This finding provides little support for the *multiple* switches that characterize the practice of many contemporary psychiatrists and primary care physicians. Again, in the absence of a control group, one cannot separate the effects of naturalistic remission from those of prescribed drugs.

The other strategy used to deal with treatment resistance is *augmentation* with other drugs. Although this option is used often, it has a surprisingly weak evidence base. Some expert reviews have concluded that the best evidence by far is for augmentation of antidepressants with lithium (Carvalho, Cavalcante, Castelo, & Lima, 2007). However, due to concern about side effects, this option is not often used.

Some physicians add a second antidepressant. Actually, little evidence supports the use of multiple antidepressants (Lam et al., 2009). If the effects of different antidepressants are more or less equivalent, why should two be better than one? The argument in favor of doing so is based on a theory that if each antidepressant has a different action at the synapse, then multiple agents should cover more neurotransmitter systems. This was also the argument used to market SNRIs such as venlafaxine, which have "dual action" on noradrenergic and serotonergic pathways, even though these agents are no more efficacious for depression than SSRIs.

Despite a weak evidence base, some antidepressants have been marketed as augmenting agents. STAR*D examined the results of augmentation of citalopram with either bupropion (currently a very popular choice) or buspirone, and it concluded that there can be a small benefit to doing so (Rush, 2007). However, because clinical trials have not confirmed these effects, the use of multiple antidepressants is of doubtful efficacy.

Augmentation with antipsychotics presents a more complex problem. Little controversy exists as to the use of antipsychotics for severe depression with melancholic and/ or psychotic features, for which they are usually necessary (Parker & Manicavasagar, 2005). The problem lies in whether antipsychotics, with all their side effects, should be prescribed to patients with mild or moderate depression. On the one hand, clinical trials have shown that antipsychotics such as quetiapine, aripiprazole, and lurasidone, when added to standard treatment with SSRIs, can increase their efficacy in depression. All three have been approved for this purpose (Kennedy, Lam, Patten, & Ravindran, 2009), but the bar set by the US Food and Drug Administration is very low (two trials, usually paid for by industry). It may make sense to use these agents on a short-term basis to control insomnia, but even then, the question of cost–benefit remains. Antipsychotics have serious side effects, and once started, patients tend to be on them for a long time. It is worth noting that rating scales, such as the Hamilton Scale for Rating Depression (Hamilton, 1960), are heavily weighted with questions about insomnia. Therefore, any agent that helps patients to sleep will show reductions on this measure, giving the false impression of a more specific effect on mood.

Another question, applicable to all of psychopharmacology, is whether to continue with the same regime when patients are remitted or when they show only a partial response. Increasingly more patients who receive drugs for depression take them for many years. Fortunately, a lifetime course of antidepressants is relatively safe. But the same is not true for atypical antipsychotics, which, even in small doses, can cause metabolic syndrome. In a systematic review, Spielmans et al. (2013) concluded,

> Atypical antipsychotic medications for the adjunctive treatment of depression are efficacious in reducing observer-rated depressive symptoms, but clinicians should interpret these findings cautiously in light of (1) the small-to-moderate-sized benefits, (2) the lack of benefit with regards to quality of life or functional impairment, and (3) the abundant evidence of potential treatment-related harm.

Similarly, in a Cochrane review, Komossa, Depping, Gaudchau, Kissling, and Leucht (2010) concluded that although the benefits of antipsychotics for depression are better than placebo, they are small and associated with diminished tolerability.

Yet atypical antipsychotics, despite their limited value and serious side effects, are being used almost routinely, particularly for insomnia, as well as for other doubtful indications. It has been suggested that antipsychotics could be used as a monotherapy for depression (Chen, Gao, & Kemp, 2011). But even at low doses, antipsychotics can produce metabolic side effects. Moreover, this kind of "augmentation" has not undergone the same meta-analytic scrutiny as has been done for antidepressants used alone. Thus, when Nelson and Papakostas (2009) favored their use (based on a meta-analysis of RCTs), in a letter, Carroll (2010) pointed out that effects are small and that no one has examined long-term outcome. That omission is par for the course in psychopharmacological research.

The long-term use of antidepressants is worrying but is relatively benign. So why would one begin treatment by prescribing a drug with serious side effects as opposed to one that does not? And if the reason for the prescription is that patients are suffering from insomnia, there are many other options.

In conjunction with a broader initiative in US medicine to support evidence-based practice ("Choosing Wisely"), the American Psychiatric Association (2015) published the following warnings:

1. Don't prescribe antipsychotic medications to patients for any indication without appropriate initial evaluation and appropriate ongoing monitoring.

2. Don't routinely prescribe two or more antipsychotic medications concurrently.
3. Don't routinely use antipsychotics as first choice to treat behavioral and psychological symptoms of dementia.
4. Don't routinely prescribe antipsychotic medications as a first-line intervention for insomnia in adults.

These are exactly the mistakes that are made by many practitioners. As documented by Olfson, Blanco, Liu, Wang, and Correll (2012), there has been a dramatic increase in the prescription of antipsychotics to patients of all ages, including children. This is not to say they should never be used for non-psychotic patients, but only that routine use for so many indications reflects a lack of consideration of cost–benefit.

THE ROAD TO POLYPHARMACY

Psychiatry today is afflicted by overly zealous prescriptions. Many of these practices are also associated with overly zealous diagnoses (Paris, 2015b). Overdiagnosis of bipolar disorder leads to increases in prescriptions of mood stabilizers as well as antipsychotics, whereas overdiagnosis of attention deficit hyperactivity disorder (ADHD) feeds the use of stimulants. One also sees more patients who are prescribed all of these agents at the same time. A large-scale survey by Kantor et al. (2015) found that the rate of polypharmacy in medical treatment as a whole increased almost twofold between 1999 and 2012.

Thus, many psychiatric patients who in the past would have received only one drug are currently being treated with polypharmacy (Mojtabai & Olfson, 2010), which is associated with a higher burden of side effects. Even when drugs are sedating, patients may receive a separate prescription for insomnia—either a benzodiazepine or, increasingly more commonly, an antipsychotic. Implausibly, the assumption is that symptoms can be separated from each other, requiring separate drugs to treat each of them.

I am often asked to consult on patients who have been given two or three drugs. But I also consult on patients who have been given six drugs, at least one from each class, with doubling of antidepressants and antipsychotics added for good measure. Surprisingly, patients do not usually rebel against these irrational practices. Some believe that the combination of so many drugs demonstrates the knowledge and skill of their treating physician.

Following the principle, "When all you have is a hammer, everything looks like a nail," psychiatrists are prescribing drugs for most of their patients. All have a proper use—one cannot treat psychosis without antipsychotics, melancholic depression without antidepressants, or bipolar disorder without mood stabilizers. But in common mental disorders, drugs have come to replace other evidence-based treatments. It is therefore not surprising that patients who receive polypharmacy are not being offered psychotherapy as an option.

In a review of the impact of psychopharmacology on psychiatry, noted researcher Baldessarini (2014) commented,

> The basic idea is that, as the science of drug action (pharmacodynamics) has made initial small advances, it has been irresistibly tempting to argue that the opposite of the drug action may be a clue to pathophysiology. Among other examples, this kind of thinking led to the dopamine excess theory of

psychotic disorders and mania based on the antidopaminergic actions of most antipsychotic antimanic drugs, to various monoamine deficiency hypotheses concerning depression and some anxiety disorders based on speculations about the norepinephrine or serotonin-potentiating actions of most antidepressants. Although such theorizing stimulated a generation of clever experimentation, findings of research aimed at testing them at the clinical level has remained inconsistent and unconvincing. ... An extension of such speculations sometimes extends into clinical practice, as diagnoses or rationales for particular treatments are presented to patients couched in concepts arising from pharmacodynamics but representing little more than neuromythology. Again, the fundamental fact is that the disorders considered to lie within the province of psychiatry remain idiopathic. (p. 403)

In summary, psychopharmacology is not based, as often claimed, on solid neuroscience. Current practice remains almost entirely empirical. We have a limited set of pharmacological tools, but somehow they work. While awaiting future breakthroughs in this form of treatment, it is advisable to remain humble.

As a psychiatrist who does a large number of consultations, I find the current situation dispiriting. Because I tend to see only patients who have *not* benefited from aggressive pharmacotherapy, it is possible that I just do not consult on those who do well on these regimes. But I doubt it. My recommendations too often are attempts to correct an almost endless panoply of misdirected and unwise practices.

The most frequent scenario concerns patients who are taking one (or often two) antidepressant without symptomatic remission but are afraid to stop. This is an unfortunate train of events, but I tend to tolerate it on the grounds that antidepressants do little harm, even when taken for years. But when patients are receiving atypical neuroleptics as well, I worry much more about long-term side effects.

Another source of misfortune for patients is misdiagnosis (Paris, 2015b). For example, I have seen many cases of personality disorders that have been maintained on lithium for years. This occurs because mood instability of any kind is conflated with hypomania.

The overprescription of stimulants is a newer problem. Some adult patients do have adult ADHD. But this condition has to begin in childhood. Ignoring the requirement for determining that a patient has a neurodevelopmental disorder, physicians are giving stimulants to people who have problems in attention that most likely derive from other sources, particularly anxiety and depression (Paris, Bhat, & Thombs, 2015). The situation is further complicated by the fact that normal people have more focus when they take amphetamines (just as they do after a cup of coffee). We do not yet know the long-term cost of these practices to adults who may be on stimulants for years or decades to come.

These practices are the price for the current belief that all mental problems can be treated by drugs, putatively backed up by neuroscience. Because I love psychiatry, it saddens me to see it misused in this way.

4

THINKING INTERACTIVELY

LINEAR VERSUS INTERACTIVE CAUSALITY

Our minds favor linear thinking, with single causes leading to single effects. Thinking interactively is much more difficult.

As we have seen, understanding mental disorders as due to chemical imbalances or abnormal neural connections is very tempting. But it is wrong to view the neural level as more "real" than measures of the mind. This kind of thinking pays lip service to psychosocial factors but loses sight of the important role that life events play in the etiology of mental disorders.

In the past, psychotherapists have been just as blindly linear in their thinking. They made broad generalizations, oversimplifying the role of life experiences, sometimes attributing all psychopathology to adverse events in childhood. In parallel with the reductionism of biological psychiatry, these models failed to consider the complexity of pathways from risk factors to outcomes.

A more scientifically valid view is that mental disorders arise from complex interactions between genetic vulnerability and psychosocial adversity (Kendler & Prescott, 2006).

Interplay between genes and environment can take several forms (Rutter, 2006). There are *epigenetic* effects, in which environmental factors suppress or activate genes. There are *gene–environment correlations*, which can be *passive* (when genes in parents influence the environment for children), *active* (when a child's temperament changes the environment), or *evocative* (when a child's temperament evokes specific reactions in other people). Finally, gene–environment interactions describe a threshold for genetic influence, and pathological outcomes are only seen under specific environmental circumstances. This "if–then" sequence is probably the most important mechanism by which genes affect the mind.

In this light, one cannot understand the effects of biology on mental illness without considering environmental stressors, and one cannot understand the impact of adverse life events without considering temperamental vulnerabilities. This "stress-diathesis" model is the foundation of development psychopathology (Ciccheti & Rogosch, 1996; Rutter, 2009).

The vast majority of people, even when stressed, do not develop mental disorders. For example, no matter how severe the stressor, post-traumatic stress disorder does not emerge in most people (Breslau, Troost, Bohnert, & Luos, 2013). In other words, the bough will not break unless it is already bent.

For all these reasons, neither a purely psychological model nor a purely biological mode is consistently predictive. Biological psychiatry goes to an extreme by dismissing life events as triggers, Whereas psychodynamic psychiatry goes to the other extreme by explaining every symptom as the result of childhood events. Psychopathology is "cooked" by a combination of temperamental vulnerability and an adverse environment.

Viewing mental disorders as chemical imbalances, or as abnormal neural connections, is a temptingly simple idea. The prestige of biological psychiatry leads clinicians to lose sight of the role of psychosocial stressors. To be fair, however, psychotherapists have oversimplified the relation of life experiences to mental disorders. Their models have failed to consider the complexity of pathways from risk factors to outcomes.

The best example is child abuse. This is a complex construct that covers enormous ground, from single incidents to multiple events creating patterns of adversity that can affect children over many years (Fergusson & Mullen, 1999). Yet misleadingly, much of this research considers childhood sexual abuse as a single variable rather than as a large and heterogeneous set of risks.

As another example, consider the currently popular emphasis on failures in attachment. This theory focuses too much on the quality of parenting, failing to consider the importance of multiple attachments (Rutter & Rutter, 1993). The construct of abnormal attachment also describes a very large set of risks that are only statistically related to an even larger set of outcomes (Cassidy & Shaver, 2016). Moreover, abnormal attachment is as much a product of temperament as experience (Kagan, 1997). By and large, although childhood adversities are risk factors for mental disorders, they fail to explain why mental disorders develop. This is because most children show a remarkable level of resilience to adversity (Rutter, 2012).

WHY PSYCHIATRY NEEDS SCIENTIFIC PSYCHOLOGY

Keeping these issues in mind should help clinicians to think *interactively*. That is why psychiatrists need to know more about psychology and why clinical psychologists need to know more about neuroscience. Unfortunately, it remains true that many clinicians, not to speak of academicians, do not take the time to learn about both domains and how they interact.

To think interactively, it helps to have a broad education in a variety of disciplines. What are the basic sciences for psychiatry? All physicians are required to take courses in biology, chemistry, and physics. A knowledge of neuroscience is obviously essential for psychiatrists. But practitioners are not required to familiarize themselves with the social sciences. That makes it seem as if neuroscience has all the "hard" data, relegating psychological and social factors to the realm of soft science or common sense.

Yet psychology is as important as neuroscience as a basic science for psychiatry. If psychiatry is concerned with disorders of the mind, then psychology, which studies normal and abnormal mental functioning, is as basic a subject as biochemistry and physiology. Psychology is also unique in being a bridge discipline between biological and social sciences. Although research in psychology sometimes draws on imaging methods, it most frequently depends on self-report or observation of behavior and mental states.

One cannot even begin to study mental processes without asking people what they are thinking, how they are feeling, and how they are behaving. Usually, the meaning of neuroscience findings can only be determined in relation to these psychological measures (self-reports or clinical ratings). Moreover, there are ways to make subjective assessments both reliable and valid. That is why research psychologists devote so much of their time to psychometrics (i.e., problems in measurement). The difference from neuroscience is that when both independent and dependent variables depend on what people say about themselves, or even on direct observation, we are in a realm without the grounding provided by biomarkers. Yet short of science-fiction scenarios of reading minds through imaging or brain recording, psychological measures are the best choice.

Familiarity with psychology would also be valuable for non-psychiatric physicians. Understanding how people think and feel is certainly of more practical use than the hoops that medical and premedical students have traditionally been put through. Many older physicians will remember wasting time in school memorizing facts that can be easily looked up, such as the Krebs cycle in biochemistry or the origins and insertions of muscles in anatomy. This tradition in medical education only proves that doctors are expected to have good rote memory.

Psychology should be part of the curriculum for residency training in psychiatry, but it usually is not. Few physicians learn that psychological research is as systematic and empirical as neuroscience. It has developed ways of assessing thought, emotion, and behavior that are as valid as brain imaging. But the reductionism underlying the mantra that mental disorders are nothing but brain disorders tends to dismiss any other way of studying the mind as "soft."

The separation of psychiatry from psychology, like the separation of psychiatry from neurology, has historical roots. Psychiatry has always traded on the respect given to medicine as a whole. But psychology, which only emerged as an academic discipline at the end of the 19th century, was initially an experimental science (Baker, 2011). In the early 20th century, it moved into practical work by developing intelligence and personality testing. Clinical psychology, originally developed as a branch of education for the handicapped, was only gradually applied to broader clinical populations. Then, during the past several decades, it has become the dominant discipline in the practice of psychotherapy.

Most research in psychology is conducted on rats or humans. Clinicians would be right to ignore most findings on rodents. You can make a rat (or a monkey) addicted to alcohol, but animals do not have psychoses, and animal models of depression are, at best, approximate. (One of my colleagues tested antidepressants on rats based on how long they would swim in a barrel of water before giving up, but I had doubts about the relevance of his research to human depression.)

Psychometrics is a branch of psychology that establishes whether assessment procedures have reliability and validity. Academic psychologists usually study people through self-report questionnaires. This method requires great attention to the accuracy of measures. Although self-report methods have limitations, they have superior stability compared to clinical ratings or interviews (which are likely to be unreliable). Moreover, psychological testing can demonstrate validity by comparing measures to data obtained in other ways.

Psychometric methods can also be applied to clinical ratings. Thus, in psychiatry, psychometrics have been applied to the validation of diagnoses—this was the special interest of Robert Spitzer, who applied these principles when developing the *Diagnostic and Statistical Manual of Mental Disorders*

(DSM) system. However, in the absence of biomarkers, the reliability of DSM-5 remains problematic, even after 35 years of work (Regier et al., 2013).

There are many domains in psychology, and the broader field can be divided into a wide range of subdisciplines. If you understand child development, you will gain insight into the precursors and onset of mental disorders. If you understand trait psychology, you will gain insight into personality disorders and the traits underlying mental illness. If you understand social psychology, you will gain a better understanding of the milieu in which mental disorders arise. Finally, if you know something about cognitive psychology, you will learn how changes in thought can affect emotions and behaviors.

Most psychiatrists know little about any of these aspects of psychology. They have even less knowledge about sociology and anthropology. A knowledge of sociology is relevant for understanding social factors in disease, as measured in epidemiological research. And the quality of social networks is a key element in developing rehabilitation programs. Anthropology is relevant for understanding the role of culture in shaping symptoms of mental disorders and their treatment. Unfortunately, the current enthusiasm for neuroscience has made the social sciences seem irrelevant to psychiatry.

NATURE, NURTURE, AND MENTAL ILLNESS

The split in psychiatry between biological and psychosocial models is part of a larger issue in science: the proverbial *nature–nurture* problem. The relationship between mind and brain is a long-standing issue in philosophy and science.

Psychiatry needs a single theory that can integrate the role of genes and environment in the etiology of mental illness. Only a few mental disorders have strictly genetic causes. Even in disorders with a strong biological component, vulnerability will only lead to symptoms in specific environments. Genes do not usually carry a direct risk for symptoms, but they determine *sensitivity* to environmental factors, both positive and negative (Belsky & Pluess, 2009). The environment can sometimes have direct effects, as shown in "natural experiments." One example concerns studies of Romanian orphans showing that children who spend long periods in an orphanage after birth tend to have deficits when followed up as adolescents (Rutter, Kumsta, Schlotz, & Sonuga-Barke, 2012). Yet most effects of the environment are modulated by genetic factors, and these interactions tend to determine whether people become exposed to adversity and how sensitive they are to adversity (Rutter, 2009).

In short, mental disorders rarely have strictly environmental causes. Adverse experiences lead most consistently to psychopathology in those who are temperamentally vulnerable (Rutter, 2012). In those who are more resilient, there may be no negative outcomes, and some people are actually "steeled" by adversity. In other words, some are thin-skinned and respond badly to adversity, whereas others are thick-skinned and more readily move on.

Sensitivity to the environment can be a problem, but it can sometimes help people to function at a better than average level (Belsky & Pluess, 2009). If one is more sensitive to *both* positive and negative experiences, one may turn out better than average in a good family but worse than average in a bad family. This mechanism, in which risk and benefit arise from the same genetic variations, helps explain why so many vulnerabilities remain in the population rather than being removed by natural selection.

The same principles can be applied to all relationships between psychological adversity and adult mental disorder. Even post-traumatic stress disorder (PTSD), a diagnosis defined as a response to adverse events, only develops in a minority of those exposed to trauma, and it is associated with a heritable vulnerability (McNally, 2003). That is why most people exposed to trauma do not develop PTSD and why those who do develop PTSD have more intense responses to stressors. In a large-scale study of twins who were war veterans (True et al., 1993), each symptom listed in the DSM as a criterion for PTSD was partially heritable.

This helps explain why people have a very high rate of resilience to life stressors, even the most severe adversities (Paris, 2000; Rutter, 2012). Earlier research on trauma and adversity assumed that psychosocial factors have a direct effect on mental illness as opposed to playing a role in gene–environment interactions. Genetic factors can even account for variance that appears to be environmental (Jang, 2005). For example, in a widely discussed book, Harris (2009) argued that *most* research in developmental psychology is difficult to interpret because it fails to control for heritable factors. Researchers can control for genetic risk by studying twins. That would be a way to determine whether relationships between life stressors and mental disorders represent correlation or causation.

Depression provides an example. The trigger for a depressive episode may be a life stressor, but susceptibility to responding with depressed mood has a moderate heritable component (Kendler & Prescott, 2006). Thus, major depression derives from a mix of biological and psychosocial risk factors, and it can be treated by pharmacotherapy, psychotherapy, or both.

In history, psychiatry has leaned either toward nature or nurture. In the past, psychiatrists were as much in love with environmental explanations of mental disorder as they are today with neuroscience. It was easy to assume that adverse life events underlie psychological symptoms. One can always come up with some kind of "formulation" that assumes that such relationships are causal.

The patients we see often have major difficulties with life tasks, such as establishing and maintaining intimate relationships and/or steady employment. These problems can reflect the effects of genes, environment, and their interactions. Thus, people with genetic vulnerability may never develop a mental disorder unless exposed to life stressors. And people exposed to the most severe life stressors may never develop a mental disorder if they have a resilient temperament.

Another problem is that many clinicians and researchers simply ask patients to remember childhood events and then examine the relationship of the past to the present, which is assumed to be causal. These methods fail to disentangle genes and environment (Harris, 2009; Rutter, 2000). Again, the glass may not break unless it has already cracked. Moreover, one cannot always assume that memories of the past are accurate, as opposed to being influenced by current distress—as they often are (Paris, 2000). Finally, cross-sectional studies, in comparison to longitudinal studies, are never sufficient to establish causality.

Another example of the complex relationship between risk and outcome is that children in the same family respond very differently to adversities such as child abuse and dysfunctional families. My research group studied the sisters of women with borderline personality disorder (BPD) and found that they rarely develop the same condition—even when they experience the same level of childhood adversity in their families (Laporte et al., 2011). But when we measured personality traits (which are approximately 50% heritable and provide a rough measure of temperament), we found that the BPD patients had a very different and much more vulnerable profile.

It is not true that psychological symptoms can usually be blamed on a bad childhood, a bad spouse, or a bad boss. But it is also not true that mental symptoms arise out of chemical imbalances that have little to do with life experiences. Rather, pathology usually arises from a "two-hit" mechanism involving interactions between adverse circumstances and temperamental vulnerability.

To understand the etiology and treatment of mental disorders, we need more than a single model, whether that is biological or psychosocial. To resolve battles between the two kinds of psychiatry, we need to claim the middle ground between nature and nurture.

ADVERSITY AND COMPLEXITY

Life adversities carry a statistical risk for the development of psychological symptoms (Rutter, 2000). This does make it possible to predict pathology from adversity or to assume adversity must have occurred whenever there is pathology. But patients who develop mental disorders are more likely than non-affected populations to have been exposed to negative life experiences (Kessler, Davis, & Kendler, 1997). Some of these risks are proximal (loss of a job or a relationship). Others are distal (dysfunctional families or child abuse). This principle applies most strongly to common mental disorders. But it also applies to severe mental disorders, which although more biological in origin, also have a relationship to psychosocial risks.

The British psychiatrist Robin Murray was one of the first researchers to conceptualize schizophrenia as a neurodevelopmental disorder related to abnormal neural connections. But Murray also led research showing that the social environment has an important influence on the risk for schizophrenia. This study (Fearon, Kirkbride, Morgan, Dazzan, & Murray, 2006) compared the prevalence of the disorder among West Indian immigrants to the United Kingdom to the prevalence in their country of origin. The results, later replicated in other immigrant groups in Europe (McKenzie & Shah, 2015), show that emigrants who live as a minority in a new country are significantly more likely to develop schizophrenia. The mechanism behind this relationship has been called "social defeat" (Cantor-Graae & Selten, 2005). This is not to say that social defeat causes schizophrenia. Rather, because genetic vulnerability to the disorder is more widely distributed in the population than frank illness, there is no direct path from temperament to symptoms, and the disorder needs to be activated by stressors.

Another line of evidence for the role of psychosocial factors has emerged from studies showing that those who eventually develop schizophrenia are more likely to report abuse and neglect in childhood and, when they do develop this illness, to have more severe symptoms (Bentall, 2010). Similar risk factors have been described in patients with bipolar disorder (Etain et al., 2013). Thus, child maltreatment is not necessarily related just to PTSD or personality disorders but, rather, can be a risk factor for all mental disorders. However, the *type* of disorder that develops in an individual is probably determined by temperamental profiles.

If psychosocial risk factors play a role in the risk for highly heritable disorders, they should play an even larger role in partially heritable disorders such as major depression. And the evidence shows that they do so. The risks for depression include common precipitants associated with life's vicissitudes, such as loss of a relationship, a job, or a social network (Kendler & Prescott, 2006).

The problem in understanding the risk for major depression is that this diagnostic construct is very broad. Major depression lacks high heritability because it is heterogeneous. with a bar set very low for diagnosis (a 2-week course for five out of nine symptoms). Severe depression, in contrast, is much more heritable (Kendler & Prescott, 2006).

The idea that all depressions are a single disorder with varying levels of severity is the source of the problem. Researchers who view severe (melancholic) depression as a separate disorder requiring different treatment have challenged this unitary model (Parker & Manicavasagar, 2005). Most research fails to make this distinction. Even if patients with mild to moderate depression have an illness that reflects biological vulnerability, most of these patients also have specific psychosocial precipitants such as losses (Kendler & Prescott, 2006).

A practical implication of the models we use is the way we interpret the lack of consistent efficacy for antidepressants in patients with mild to moderate symptoms (Kirsch et al.,

2008). Many of these patients do better with psychotherapy (Beck, 2008). It makes sense that even if one is reacting more severely than expected to a recent loss or life adversity, talking about what happened may be more effective than taking medication for symptoms. (Of course, many patients do both.)

Similar considerations apply to other common mental disorders. A good example is generalized anxiety disorder (GAD; Stevens, Jendrusina, Sarapas, & Behar, 2014). Like major depression (with which it can often be comorbid), GAD is a syndrome with multiple causes, with interactions between a heritable anxious temperament and psychosocial stressors. Similarly, panic disorder can be conceptualized as a vulnerability to specific symptoms that is activated by life events (Schmidt, Korte, Norr, Keough, & Timpano, 2014).

Using a model in which disorders arise from gene–environment interactions is particularly relevant for conditions can be treated with psychotherapy and/or rehabilitation. Substance use is an example. Alcoholism is known to be heritable, with genes accounting for 50–60% of the variance (Kendler & Prescott, 2006). However, treatment, even when there is a high genetic risk, usually consists of detoxification followed by psychotherapy and group support to maintain abstinence.

Eating disorders (Thornton et al., 2010) also have a moderate heritable component (approximately 50% of the variance) and develop due to environmental risks, some of which are specific to the patient's life experience, whereas others derive from society (e.g., a preoccupation with thinness). Treatment for eating disorders is generally psychotherapeutic, designed to correct an abnormal body image.

Personality disorders, also traditionally thought to be environmental in origin, have been shown in twin studies to have a heritability close to 50% (Torgersen et al., 2000). This level of genetic vulnerability also applies to categories in which childhood adversities have been extensively studied, such as borderline and antisocial personality. Psychological risks often include family dysfunction, abuse, and neglect (Paris, 2015b) but describe no direct pathway from any risk factor to a diagnosable disorder.

An illusion of causality can emerge from seeing patients with a traumatic history and attributing adult symptoms to these adversities. What we forget is that many people experience the same traumas but never need to see us. These interactions best fit into a *biopsychosocial* model (discussed in Chapter 5).

Research on *epigenetic* mechanisms (Meaney & Szyf, 2005) shows that stressful life events can affect switching mechanisms associated with the genome (largely through a process of methylation that suppresses the activity of alleles). Thus, epigenetic theory suggests that environmental influences can change biology. Moreover, epigenetic changes can be passed on across several generations. In addition, life experiences, both positive and negative, can change connections in the brain—a concept called *neuroplasticity* (Ruge, Liou, & Hoad, 2012). Thus, learning can also change transmission in the brain, or, as it has been said, "what fires together, wires together."

It has required this kind of sophisticated research to convince some biological psychiatrists that the environment plays *any* role in development. Still, we do not know the strength of these effects or precisely how they are involved in pathways to mental disorders.

CLINICAL IMPLICATIONS
OF INTERACTIVE MODELS

Physicians, like almost everyone else, have trouble thinking in terms of multiple and interacting pathways to causation. Yet only a few conditions in medicine (e.g., some infections) follow a simple road from risk to illness. Models that acknowledge complexity are needed for chronic diseases and are especially applicable to psychiatry.

We tend to think that disorders with biological causes need biological treatment and that only disorders with a psychosocial etiology require psychotherapy. That is not true. For example, entirely genetic diseases in medicine can sometimes be treated with diet, as in the rare condition of phenylketonuria and in the common condition of diabetes type II. In psychiatry, diet and exercise can also be helpful for depression (Murphy, Straebler, Cooper, & Fairburn, 2010). And psychotherapy can still be useful in disorders known to have strong biological basis.

The best example is schizophrenia. We are not talking about long-discredited attempts to talk patients out of psychosis. Rather, a modified form of CBT, focusing on raising a certain level of doubt about delusional beliefs and developing better social skills, has been shown to be effective (Tarrier, 2005). (This was one benefit of a recent policy of the National Health Service in the United Kingdom to hire more psychologists.) But the most important implications are for common mental disorders. Anxiety and depression are often treated with drugs alone, but they are also the primary targets for psychotherapy, as shown by an enormous research literature (Lambert, 2013).

British child psychiatrist Michael Rutter (1933–), a prolific writer on gene–environment relationships, emphasizes that genes and environment are never really separate (Rutter, 2009). You cannot simply add up their effects because genes and environment constantly interact. Thus, when you assess the impact of psychosocial risk factors, what you are actually measuring is how experience was perceived and processed. Moreover, people select and shape their environments. For example, although adolescents are at higher risk if they join pathological peer groups, their personal traits lead them to choose these friends.

It follows that we cannot evaluate biological risk outside a psychosocial context. Nor can we evaluate psychosocial risks outside a context of genetic vulnerability. This is why formulations that assume cause and effect relationships between life adversity and symptoms are at best inadequate and usually wrong.

Even if the impact of psychosocial risk factors cannot be understood without considering individual differences in vulnerability, the psychiatrist's task is still to take a detailed life history. Biological psychiatry often tends to consider the past superficially, focusing primarily on family history for specific disorders.

There are several reasons why a life history is important. First, past events lead to a *sensitization* to later events. In a community study of PTSD, Breslau, Chilcoat, Kessler, and Davis (1999) showed that vulnerability (measured by trait neuroticism) as well as a history of past trauma were the best predictors of this condition. This is the same mechanism by which child adversity can sensitize people to adverse events in adulthood.

Second, past events can create patterns of dysfunction that persist over time. This failure to learn more appropriate skills (associated with resilience) may be reinforced by choosing pathological partners and peer groups (Rutter, 2012).

Third, failure to take a life history can be associated with a rush to prescribe, leading to unnecessarily aggressive pharmacological interventions (Carlat, 2010). This kind of practice has become all too common.

Finally, life stories create a *narrative*, and psychotherapy is, among other things, designed to change personal narratives. The trajectory of a problematic life has to be understood before it can be modified. Whether one calls these phenomena psychodynamics or schema, therapists work to make patients aware of them, to take ownership of their own lives, and to view themselves not as victims but as capable of changing their fate.

5

PARADIGMS AND PRACTICE

THE BIOPSYCHOSOCIAL MODEL

George Engel (1913–1999) was an American psychiatrist who had an ambitious goal: to develop a general theory of illness and healing in medicine. His *biopsychosocial* (BPS) model (Engel, 1980) was directed toward all medical practitioners, but it has been most often applied to psychiatry, family medicine, and health psychology. A BPS approach takes a broad view of etiology, considering the influence of heritable vulnerabilities, psychological adversities, and social stressors. As a *systems theory*, BPS contrasts with reductionist models that attempt to explain complex phenomena by reducing them to simpler components. BPS also takes a broad view of treatment, supporting a multimodal approach to medical treatment. It therefore stands in contrast to the strictly *biomedical* model used in most areas of medicine, including modern psychiatry.

In proposing this model, Engel hoped to change attitudes among physicians and to make them more sensitive to psychosocial factors in illness. However, he did not anticipate the extent to which the march of technology would reinforce a biomedical model. Approximately 30 years ago, most psychiatrists were still using psychotherapy, and neuroscience had only begun its progress. Today, although many physicians and psychiatrists pay lip service to BPS, it does not guide research or practice (Borrell-Carrio, Suchman, & Epstein, 2004).

It is also rare to see research in psychiatry that measures biological and psychosocial risk factors in the same population. A famous exception is the well-known studies by Caspi et al. (2002, 2003), in which an interaction between genetic variants (affecting neurotransmitter activity) and childhood adversities (e.g., a history of abuse) influenced the risk for antisocial personality as well as for depression. Yet by and large, biological research remains biological, and psychosocial research remains psychosocial.

Critics of the BPS model tend to prefer a biomedical approach. Ghaemi (2010) considered BPS to be a fuzzy concept leading to mere eclecticism. McLaren (1998) viewed BPS as less of a predictive model than a general point of view that is not sufficiently precise to drive research. It is true that a simplistic view of Engel's model could involve just adding up a list of risks from different sources. But there is no reason why BPS could not be applied as a predictive model to describe complex interactions. This is why statistical analysis in many papers published today uses regression methods and hierarchical linear modeling, in which multiple independent variables can be assessed in relation to a range of outcomes.

In principle, BPS should be vastly superior to the purely biomedical approach that Bentall (2010) calls a "bio-bio-bio" model. But for clinicians, thinking about patients in a BPS model in practice is a challenge. The human mind is programmed to view cause and effect in linear relationships (Pinker, 1997). It is very tempting to seize on a single risk factor as an explanation for a clinical outcome. It is much more difficult to understand mental disorders using an interactive model. One has to consider both the biological factors that lead to vulnerability and the adverse experiences that activate pathological mechanisms. Even so, if properly applied, BPS could be a research tool and an important counter to dismissive attitudes toward psychosocial psychiatry.

Why, then, has BPS failed to become the primary paradigm for psychiatry? Largely, this is because it was overtaken by the triumphal march of neuroscience. Reviewing the status of the model 15 years ago, Pilgrim (2002) concluded that BPS remained well outside the mainstream. There is little reason to think that this situation has changed since then.

A failure to be multimodal affects all aspects of psychiatry. I have discussed the tendency of biological psychiatry to minimize the effects of the environment. I have also noted that most psychosocial approaches show scant awareness of biology and rarely take temperamental vulnerability into account. The social psychiatry of the 1960s, with its grandiose claim that psychiatrists could change society, was a particularly egregious example.

Thus, I do not advocate returning to the bad old days when purely psychological models dominated psychiatry. The result sometimes led to blaming parents for every problem. I lived through those times. Patients and their families suffered unnecessarily. Moreover, many (if not most) patients were told they needed long-term psychotherapy, even though there was no empirical support for such a recommendation. Now we have gone to the other extreme, blaming neurotransmitters and connectivity for every mental disorder. Moreover, every patient is given a prescription, with or without supporting evidence. It seems difficult for most clinicians to take an integrated and interactive perspective, for which no better word than "biopsychosocial" has yet been found.

In summary, the BPS model has not been adopted because it is too complicated and because we live in an age of adulation for neuroscience. The pharmaceutical industry has convinced the public that depression and anxiety are due to a chemical imbalance that can be corrected by a pill. Psychotherapy is difficult to access and often not even considered in cases in which it has been shown to be effective.

Yet current practice might change if consumers were to demand access to a wider range of treatments. Many patients today have the same perceptions as their physicians—that neuronal pathways and chemistry explain the origins of mental disorders. Their impression is that pharmacological treatment is scientific, that talking therapy is not, and that psychological problems are best treated by drugs. There will always be patients who do not see the point of talking about problems, either for psychological or for cultural reasons. Yet surveys show that a majority still want psychotherapy (McHugh, Whitton, Peckham, Welge, & Ottos, 2013). Most patients would welcome adding psychotherapy to their treatment package—if only it was easily available.

DSM DIAGNOSIS AND ITS ILLUSIONS

Psychiatry began in the asylum, where patients were so sick that it was not difficult to distinguish their symptoms from problems in living that occur in normal people. The situation changed when specialists moved into office practice. There has never been a clear boundary between unhappiness and depression (Horwitz & Wakefield, 2007) or between fear and anxiety (Horwitz & Wakefield, 2011). Some suspect that what therapists really want is to work with normal people. For this reason, psychiatrists who practice only psychotherapy have been accused of treating the "worried well."

Although psychiatry has tried to make diagnosis more precise, it cannot achieve this goal in the absence of biomarkers. Until the 1970s, psychiatry had a classification of mental disorders that was vague and that was not a useful guide to practice. But as long as leaders in the field were psychoanalysts, diagnosis was not taken seriously. This left psychiatry open to attack. Other specialties, as well as other mental health professions, viewed the diagnosis of mental disorders with skepticism. Psychiatry rightly became worried about the specialty's legitimacy within medicine (Decker, 2013).

Melvin Sabshin, who headed the American Psychiatric Association from 1974 to 1997, set out to redress this problem by appointing a task force to recommend revision of the classification of mental disorders. This process led to the publication of the third edition of the *Diagnostic and Statistical Manual of Mental Disorders* (DSM-III; American Psychiatric Association, 1980). The manual aimed to be theoretically neutral to avoid the errors of previous editions, which used psychoanalytic concepts such as "unconscious conflict" to support diagnostic entities. But by using symptoms, independent of life circumstances, as criteria for diagnoses, DSM-III implicitly promoted biological psychiatry. Symptoms are easier to view as targets for modification by drugs.

Even if this was not the intention, the DSM manuals are partly responsible for patterns of overdiagnosis and overtreatment (Paris, 2015b). Instead of delineating its scope more precisely, psychiatry has chosen to create manuals of mental disorders that reflect what practitioners do and that can be used to justify treating almost any human problem.

The DSM system was introduced to make psychiatry more scientific, and in some ways, it succeeded. However, that does not mean that the diagnoses listed in the manual are based on solid empirical data. It is just the best we can do for now (Paris, 2015a). With constant use during approximately the past 35 years, the system has become reified and essential to the worldview of psychiatry. DSM diagnoses are actually little but shorthand terms to describe syndromes. They remain useful for communication. But most categories will not survive in the long term. In the future, the DSM manual may be regarded as a relic of an earlier era, in which the causes of mental disorders were not yet understood.

Biological psychiatrists like to believe they are treating categories of illness as real as tuberculosis and that the drugs they use are as specific and scientifically grounded as antibiotics. They are wrong on both counts. We use categories in science because they help us communicate and because our minds are programmed to think that way. The real world is more complex than we think or can even imagine.

Many scientific categories are fuzzy around the edges. Species in biology are a good example. Although long-separated populations become separate when they can no longer interbreed, a large number of intermediates must have existed in the course of their evolution. In this way, quantitative differences can become qualitative.

Medicine has always viewed illness as categorical and has searched for treatments that are specific to diagnoses. Its greatest triumphs have been in infectious diseases, in which treatment methods are based on the causes of disease. The idea that diagnosis leads directly to treatment reflects success in that domain. (Even so, complex immunological mechanisms determine who falls ill and who does not.) But this scenario does not apply to chronic diseases with a complex etiology, in which the mechanisms that lead to disease are multivariate and interactive.

In psychiatry, despite our ignorance, the medications we prescribe help most patients, and our treatments stand up well in comparison to those of other specialties (Leucht, Hierl, Kissling, Dold, & Davis, 2012). But we are a long way from specificity. We know little about the causes of most of the illnesses we treat. Moreover, many, if not most, mental disorders are chronic, with a complex etiology.

The DSM system attempted to avoid premature conclusions by postponing etiological explanations and by focusing on thorough and reliable clinical observation. But it failed to define the endophenotypes that can be targets for treatment. For this reason, critics of the DSM system, such as Thomas Insel (2015), have viewed it as unscientific. But we lack a good alternative.

As discussed in Chapter 1, Insel (2015) was instrumental in developing the Research Domain Criteria (RDoC) system that offers to replace DSM diagnoses with a matrix of scores on biological measures. RDoC proponents are wildly optimistic about its ability to cut nature at its joints. But at this point, it has little better to offer than DSM (Paris & Kirmayer, 2016). It may be unscientific to describe disorders entirely on the basis of their symptoms, but it is no less unscientific to define them based on a raw and undeveloped neurobiology.

The best example of diagnostic reification in the DSM system is major depressive disorder (MDD). This is, of course, the most common diagnosis in clinical practice. But as a student, I was taught that depression can be a symptom, a syndrome, or an illness. Since DSM-III was published in 1980, MDD has become a single category of disease with a spectrum of severity. This has led to a perception that MDD is one diagnosis responding to one type of pharmacological treatment. When physicians state, "This patient has a major depression," you can be sure they are already reaching for their prescription pads.

Yet MDD is not even reliable from one clinician to another (Regier et al., 2013). More than 35 years after DSM-III, we have reified this diagnosis. MDD is a label of some practical value for describing a heterogeneous group of patients, but it should not be treated as a disease. I have no problem with using MDD as a shorthand term for a syndrome. I do have a problem when every depressed patient, no matter what the cause of morbidity, is treated with antidepressants.

These comments apply to mild and moderate depression but exclude severe depression (melancholia), in which pharmacological treatment is absolutely essential. The mild to moderate end of the spectrum is where the problem lies. After decades of practice, I still have difficulty understanding what the difference is between unhappiness and mild depression. I have also lived long enough to know that life offers a fair share of unhappiness to most of us. This helps explain the high lifetime prevalence of MDD (Kessler et al., 2005)— 13% in men and 21% in women. We respond with sadness to life's adversities, which often produce depressive symptoms. Some have even thought that a temporarily lowered mood is an adaptation that can help people cope with adversity (Nesse, 2005).

I have no hesitation in prescribing drugs for patients who are severely depressed—that is, unable to sleep or unable to work. I agree with many colleagues that the best treatments for melancholia are antidepressants, antipsychotics, and electroconvulsive therapy. But the majority of patients do not have such severe symptoms. That is why treating all depression as one disease, to be treated with the same medications, makes little sense. An overly broad category leads inevitably to overtreatment.

Also, diagnosing major depression does not necessarily mean that the disorder afflicts patients who would otherwise be healthy. Zimmerman et al. (2008) found that approximately half of all patients attending outpatient clinics, most of whom meet criteria for MDD, meet criteria for a preexisting personality disorder (PD). Even if one does not believe in the existence of PDs (some biological psychiatrists do not), these data nonetheless show that many of the patients who see psychiatrists for depression have had serious life problems for many years. They are not normal people afflicted by a reversible biological error. Their depression is part of their life and their personality.

THE RISE OF THE 15-MINUTE MED CHECK

Surveys document that psychiatrists are spending less time with each patient and providing less psychotherapy than they did in the past. Mojtabai and Olfson (2008) reported that the percentage of visits with at least 30 minutes of psychotherapy decreased over a 10-year period from 44% to 29%. This retreat from the 50-minute hour might be less of a problem if it were easy to refer patients to other professionals for psychological treatment. But doing so is not easy. Psychologists and social workers provide services but are inadequately insured. Most of the patients I consult on cannot afford to pay fees out of pocket, and they also lack good insurance coverage. The result is that even though psychotherapy is as evidence-based and cost-effective as many other treatments, patients who can benefit from it are not receiving it. This may be due to the stigma attached to psychological problems, as well as the reputation of psychotherapy for being interminable, which makes insurers reluctant to cover it.

Today, much of psychiatric practice has come to consist of these *med checks*. Not much has been written on this subject. But a journalist, Gardiner Harris, discussed the problem in 2011 in an article titled "Talk Doesn't Pay, So Psychiatry Turns Instead to Drug Therapy." The focus was on a psychiatrist who used to do therapy but gave up seeing any patients for an hour, opting instead to do nothing but review medication for hundreds of people.

It has now become common for psychiatrists to offer many of their patients 15-minute sessions (Gabbard, 2009). Needless to say, the focus of these meetings is on pharmacology. In this kind of practice, all patients receive medication—and *only* medication. Assessments on each visit may also make use of a checklist, which in turn will be based on criteria for their diagnosis listed in the DSM manual. (The various editions of DSM have made a point of stating that its criteria are not designed to guide treatment choices, but few clinicians pay much attention to that warning.) Within a limited time frame, all one can do is to inquire about the reasons for changes in current symptoms, focusing on DSM criteria. If patients are feeling worse, they get a change of medication—either an increased dose or a new drug. If they are feeling the same or better, they are advised to continue the same treatment. It almost never happens that patients are advised to stop medication or to try psychotherapy.

Psychiatrists who practice in this way have no time to be interested in the psychosocial factors that drive symptoms. They are not in a position to view patients as people with life stories or as collaborators who can play an active role in their own recovery. Instead, patients are seen as passive recipients of treatments designed to change aberrant neurochemistry. Perhaps clinicians who practice in this way believe that psychosocial aspects of illness are irrelevant. This is the "bio-bio-bio" model in action (Bentall, 2010). Or as one psychiatrist (Markowitz, 2016) stated in an op-ed, there can be too much neuroscience.

I have not painted a pretty picture, but psychiatrists are doing what pays best and what best fits the paradigm they are using. By prescribing medication for every life problem or symptom, they are applying the tools they have been trained to use and with which they are most familiar.

Of course, drugs for anxiety and depression can still be a useful option. But it does not follow that every patient with these symptoms should receive them. The idea that depressed patients can be treated without drugs is difficult to support if one uses the guidelines published by the American Psychiatric Association (2010), which considers pharmacology as the first line of intervention, no matter what the cause of the depression. In contrast, initial follow-up of patients *without* immediate pharmacological interventions is a prominent feature of the British guideline published by the National Institute for Care Excellence (2009).

In a biomedical model, antidepressants are viewed, much like antibiotics, as specific treatments with predictable results. When patients get better, for any reason (e.g., a placebo response or a change in life circumstances), drugs are given the credit. If they do not work, then it is assumed that the patient is "treatment resistant" and requires more aggressive interventions.

The med check is also the default mode of treatment in primary care. Non-psychiatric physicians are now more comfortable prescribing than they used to be—partly due to better education and partly due to better side effect profiles. But not everyone takes the trouble to follow patients closely during the crucial first few weeks of treatment. Instead, initial prescriptions may be written for a month and sometimes even include a request to the pharmacy for repeats. Yet antidepressants should be initially prescribed for a week to allow for close monitoring in the early stages of treatment. Specific serotonin reuptake inhibitors and serotonin–noradrenaline reuptake inhibitors can have troublesome side effects and also take time to work, so prescribing them without careful follow-up is a recipe for noncompliance and ineffective treatment.

Physicians who are not even in a position to follow patients may still prescribe antidepressants. This can happen in a crisis presenting in the emergency room or in primary care settings that allow for drop-ins. If a patient is psychotic, or if the situation is relatively urgent, it may make sense to send patients home with a small dose of an appropriate drug. But given the evidence that results are slow to emerge and are also inconsistent in mild to moderate depression, many patients are being prescribed medication they do not need—and may not even take. Again, the side effects that cause so many to stop taking these drugs are the reason why new prescriptions need close follow-up.

Moreover, patients are not necessarily given the option of opting for psychotherapy instead of drugs. Nor is therapy considered an option for those who do not (or only partially) respond to medication. Instead, depressed patients are routinely offered additional drugs, leading to a practice marked by polypharmacy. Some of them end up on five drugs or more.

How did this parody of treatment come to dominate practice? The most obvious reason is that psychiatrists make more money by seeing four patients in 1 hour instead of one patient. Insurance, whether it comes from governments or from private sources, does not favor 50-minute hours.

A deeper reason has to do with the identity of the specialty. Psychiatry wants to be like the rest of medicine and to gain the same respect accorded other physicians. It does not want to be viewed as a variant of clinical psychology but, rather, as a medical discipline conducting scientific diagnosis and treatment.

The older image of a psychiatrist, as a psychoanalyst who looks deep into the human soul, has become an anachronism. It has been replaced by the image of an expert psychopharmacologist who knows how to mix and match the latest medications, based on neuroscience data defining specific effects on neurotransmitter sites. Actually, a practice exclusively based on psychopharmacology is neither evidence-based nor consistently effective.

Most psychiatrists know far too little about the strong scientific evidence for the efficacy of psychotherapy. It can be as evidence-based as is psychopharmacology is (or pretends to be). They also are not aware of the cost–benefit and practicability of this treatment. (These issues are examined in Chapter 6.) By adopting a narrow biological model, psychiatry has given up much of what has made it valuable and unique.

I am not a psychiatrist who wants to go back to the "good old days." (I lived through those days, and they were not particularly good.) But some people feel differently. For example, Tanya Luhrmann, an anthropologist who writes columns for *The New York Times* and whose father was a psychoanalyst, wrote a book titled *Of Two Minds* (Luhrmann, 2000), highlighting the split between biological psychiatry and psychotherapy in resident training. But Luhrmann waxed nostalgic about a past psychiatry that suffered from a set of problems at least as bad as the ones we face today. Patients received treatments that were not evidence-based and that could go on for years. The result was a waste of precious time—both for consumers and for professionals.

WHY PSYCHIATRY REMAINS MYSTERIOUS

Physicians in other medical specialties still find psychiatry mystifying. The idea that one might spend time talking to patients (rather than prescribing drugs) can seem strange and alien. When I was a student, professors of medicine discouraged their students from choosing psychiatry as a profession. This situation has not changed much throughout the years. I still hear about teachers whose response to the choice of psychiatry is "But I thought you were smart." If this attitude is so common, we need to ask why.

The most important reason is stigma (Corrigan, 2005). *Everyone* is afraid of mental illness. People are understandably concerned about having any condition in which they are not in control of their own minds. For that reason, mental illness has always been the subject of defensive humor—at least until the humorist (or a member of the humorist's family) develops a serious problem. Thus, even as psychiatry can be dismissed, it can also be feared. (It is the only medical specialty that has been opposed by a movement describing itself as "antipsychiatry.")

Psychiatry was born in mental hospitals, places where most patients were severely ill (and often admitted involuntarily). But over time, most practice came to be conducted in offices and outpatient settings (Shorter, 1997). These psychiatrists spent more time treating common mental disorders, for which psychotherapy is most appropriate. But today, practitioners view these conditions as indications for pharmacological management.

Some disorders that psychiatrists see are difficult to manage without medical skills, particularly when symptoms are severe. Addictions are a good example, and this is one reason why patients with more severe substance abuse tend to benefit from specialized clinics (Rush, McPherson-Does, Behroozm, & Cudmore, 2013). Similar considerations apply to severe cases of eating disorder (Wilson, Vitousek, & Loeb, 2000). In recent decades, we have learned that patients with severe personality disorders benefit most from specific methods of psychotherapy (Paris, 2015a). But because these patients see physicians first, they tend to be unnecessarily treated with drugs. There are times when the skills of a psychiatrist in prescribing these agents are definitely needed, but many cases of personality disorder can be treated with psychotherapy alone.

Despite extensive research on the efficacy of psychotherapy, the critical view of psychiatry held by other physicians continues to be based on skepticism about "talking cures." Psychiatrists feel more comfortable doing what other physicians do—making diagnoses and prescribing medication. Patients often ask, "How can *talking* help?" Quite a few psychiatrists have thought it cannot. The skeptics are now in the majority.

PSYCHIATRY CHANGES ITS PARADIGM

When I was a resident, psychiatry prided itself on its eclecticism. Biological methods were predominant in hospitals, where most patients had conditions that required medication and benefited little from talking. Psychosocial methods were most predominant in office practice, where medication was viewed as having only marginal value.

In medicine, paradigms determine practice. Two kinds of psychiatry created two kinds of psychiatrists. Prior to World War II, psychotherapists were a minority. But in the post-war period, psychoanalysis gained a dominant influence on academic psychiatry in North America, and many department chairs identified themselves primarily as analysts. That trend created the image of psychiatry that has long fascinated humorists, as shown by cartoons of analysts treating patients on the couch published over many decades in *The New Yorker*.

But if psychiatrists were *only* psychotherapists, why would they need to have an MD? (Even today, psychoanalysts tend to refer patients elsewhere for prescriptions.) One can reasonably ask whether psychiatrists who only do therapy are "real doctors" or clinical psychologists with a different degree. This is the gap between psychiatry and medicine that biological models aimed to close.

Effective drugs were crucial in making biological psychiatry the dominant paradigm for the field. Prior to the 1950s, pharmacological treatments were not very effective. Then a series of dramatic breakthroughs occurred that impressed everyone, as I saw during my own training. No psychotherapist could claim to pull patients out of a psychosis or a severe depression within weeks or days—but drugs could.

The problem was that drugs originally developed for useful purposes were gradually used for a wider range of patients. Slowly but surely, antidepressants (often combined with antipsychotics as augmenting agents) began to be prescribed routinely for patients with common mental disorders. These developments have been applauded by their advocates as bringing psychiatry back into the mainstream of medicine. I am not that impressed, and I have serious questions about the evidence behind these prescriptions. Moreover, practice cannot be strongly scientific when so little is known about the brain.

Another reason for the return to a biomedical model was the rise of evidence-based medicine (EBM; Evidence-Based Medicine Working Group, 1992). During the next few decades, this movement gained momentum and became a paradigm shift. Top journals now only published empirical data, and editors would not even look at papers that depended primarily on clinical observation. It was also no longer possible for clinicians without data-based publications to obtain leadership positions in academia. Biological psychiatrists, some of whom had published hundreds of these papers, were happy to fill that niche.

This shift was, in many ways, progressive. You cannot prove much by speculating, particularly about the meaning of what patients say to therapists. Psychiatry joined the EBM movement and prided itself on promoting evidence-based practice, measurement, and randomized controlled trials of treatment.

It is understandable that psychiatry wants to be recognized as legitimate. But despite the miracles that can occur with biological treatment for severe mental disorders, these models are much less appropriate for common mental disorders. Even if we accept the view that advances in neuroscience will eventually explain more about mental illness, the complexity of this task makes it a project for a century.

Moreover, it is not necessary for psychiatry to be totally biological in order to be scientific or legitimate. Some of the most important findings in the field have had nothing to do with biology or chemistry. For example, research on the long-term effects of childhood adversity has learned enormously from the prospective follow-up of cohorts from childhood to adulthood (Rutter, 2000). And evidence for the effectiveness of psychotherapy can be collected without identifying genes or biomarkers.

Yet although research on psychological treatment, as well as meta-analyses of this research, has sometimes been published in top journals such as *JAMA Psychiatry* or the *American Journal of Psychiatry*, these publications have been exceptional. One can easily find results of psychological research in reports from the Cochrane Collaboration, but psychiatrists only rarely consult that authoritative source. Psychiatrists who attend conferences promoting continuing medical education will only hear about pharmacotherapy.

These events are usually paid for by the pharmaceutical industry, which promotes its own agenda.

One result is that psychology and psychiatry, once partners, have fallen out of synch. Psychologists continue to practice their own craft, guided by the books and workshops used to promote psychotherapy. Even so, intimidated by claims for the latest drugs, they may send their patients to psychiatrists (or primary care physicians) to assess suitability for pharmacotherapy—with the result that many, if not most, receive prescriptions on top of psychological treatment.

THE CURRENT STATE OF PSYCHIATRY

Armed with a biological paradigm, psychiatry now attracts a different type of student. When I graduated in 1964, 10% of my class elected to train in psychiatry. At the time, this high frequency of choice for psychiatry was not unusual throughout North America. In those days, few went into family medicine, so for students who aspired to be humanistic, psychiatry was the best choice. (Action-oriented students usually preferred surgery, whereas deeper thinkers usually chose internal medicine.)

Today, psychiatry attracts only 2% or 3% of medical graduates (Lyons, 2013). Paradoxically, this may be because the specialty is less unique. Fewer of its practitioners spend much time practicing any formal form of psychotherapy. Those who want to focus on psychological interventions might be better advised to take a PhD in clinical psychology. Even so, modern psychiatry still attracts students fascinated with the mystery of severe mental illness who also want to develop better ways of treating it. (This was my primary motivation to choose the specialty.) Even so, trainees quickly discover that the main paradigm today is neuroscience.

In retrospect, the psychopharmacological revolution was an inspiring era to study psychiatry. Patients formerly considered to be hopelessly ill recovered and were discharged into the community. Even if the results were not always as good as we hoped, I agree with David Healy (1997) that this was a great moment in the history of medicine.

Yet these miracles came at a price. The main one was overconfidence. Our tools were powerful but not powerful enough to help all patients. Yet with the encouragement of the pharmaceutical industry and of academics specializing in psychopharmacology, it was widely believed that experts had unique skills to mix and match the latest drugs. This was reminiscent of what happened when psychiatrists discovered that psychoanalysis was limited in efficacy—its advocates argued that it was not the method that was wrong but, rather, lack of skill of those who used it.

During the past several decades, although many new drugs have been developed, they are hardly more effective than older ones. Most are "me-too" agents that are good enough to be approved by regulators but have no unique benefits. Moreover, psychiatrists greatly overestimate the efficacy of the drugs they prescribe. These misperceptions have been supported by academics in the pay of industry, as well as by physicians who depend entirely on pharmaceutical representatives to update their knowledge (Frances, 2013). Yet psychiatrists have been reluctant to accept that antidepressants are less consistently effective than most practitioners think.

Meanwhile, many psychiatrists are unaware that psychotherapy is a practical and evidence-based option for the treatment of common mental disorders. One reason is that empirical findings on efficacy tend to appear in psychology journals that they do not read. A second reason is that there is no equivalent for psychotherapy of pharmaceutical representatives and academic pharmacologists, who have done so much to convince psychiatrists that drugs can work for almost everyone. Instead, psychotherapy has to be promoted by psychologists who write books (that psychiatrists also do not read). A third reason is the culture of psychiatry within medicine. The leading teachers of the next generation are biologically oriented. Finally, psychoanalysis retains a strong role in some universities. Where I work, many of the psychiatrists who teach psychotherapy to psychiatrists in training are psychoanalysts without a serious commitment to evidence-based practice.

One current problem in teaching psychiatry is that skills in interviewing are no longer valued in the same way. Even psychiatrists who do not practice formal therapy need to know how to talk to patients. The American surgeon Atul Gawande (2014) has described how he discovered that talking to patients about their impending death was as much of a "procedure" as an operation. There is equally good evidence to conclude that psychotherapy is a technique that does not come naturally but has to be learned.

The practice of psychiatry has changed since the heyday of psychoanalysis, when the "50-minute hour" was standard. That length of time was sufficient for formal psychotherapy, as well as for the writing of prescriptions. But that kind of practice has dwindled as the 15-minute medication check became standard. This time frame is too brief to allow for psychological interventions, but it is used to conduct an inventory of symptoms and to determine whether current medication should be altered or changed. This kind of practice deviates so far from evidence-based medicine that it can only be called a travesty.

Med checks may well be sufficient to manage chronic patients with severe mental disorders who are reasonably stable, but they are insufficient for the treatment of most common mental disorders. In these cases, one needs to take the time to find out what is going on in the patient's life. When there are recent life stressors, it is often more important to identify and address them than to increase or change a prescription.

Current practice is sometimes based on psychopharmacological algorithms. Thus, if a patient fails to respond to an antidepressant, the dose can be increased, a second antidepressant can be added, or an augmenting agent can be prescribed. Although these procedures sometimes work, they often do not. The evidence on which these algorithms is based is weak. The problem is that medications lack the specificity and clinical efficacy we would like. Meta-analyses have provided evidence that antidepressants are not always better than placebo for mild to moderate depression, that most antidepressants have similar levels of efficacy, that the use of multiple antidepressants has a weak evidence base, and that augmenting agents may do little more than add sedation (Healy, 2002). The truth is that there is insufficient evidence to build reliable and valid algorithms for the treatment of any mental disorder. When you look at them closely, you will be surprised to learn how weak the evidence is for each step (Paris, 2010a).

Moreover, psychopharmacology is based on a model that targets symptoms, not people. It is only when one moves beyond symptomatic assessment, and looks at the person being treated, that other options become possible. One of these options is psychotherapy, if provided in a brief time frame, which can help many patients who do not respond to drugs.

Unfortunately, there is little point in recommending a treatment that is unavailable. Psychiatrists, even those who are interested in therapy, are not always fully trained to carry out these procedures themselves. Outside of the medical system, large numbers of practicing psychologists are looking for this kind of work. Not all of them have received a rigorous training in therapy. But even if they have, patients often cannot pay their fees. Insurance companies are suspicious of supporting what they fear will turn out to be long-term therapy, and they usually pay for only a few crisis sessions—less than what research shows to be a minimum. These problems of access to effective treatment need to be addressed by the mental health system.

I can remember a time when drugs were just becoming standard for schizophrenia and bipolar disorder. These agents helped millions to recover from serious mental illness. But those advances were not translated into effective treatment for common mental disorders. That is why I would like to see psychiatry return to its biopsychosocial roots. This model states that if the causes of mental illness are biological, psychological, and social, then treatments should be similarly broad and eclectic. I am arguing for a practice that gives patients the time to talk about their lives and to be heard. The results would be better than what we have now.

6

WHAT PSYCHIATRISTS DO NOT
KNOW ABOUT PSYCHOTHERAPY

PSYCHOTHERAPY RESEARCH

Unlike pharmacological interventions, which focus on symptoms, psychotherapy aims to modify mental processes. Yet even though the research base for psychological treatment is as good as that for most drugs, many psychiatrists do not know enough about it. Psychotherapy is not featured in the journals they read or in continuing medical education. Needless to say, pharmaceutical representatives never come to the door promoting it. If they read more, academics may have a better appreciation of this option. But those who do not know the literature may view psychotherapy as a fuzzy subject. If psychiatrists believed that patients would benefit from psychotherapy, they would offer it themselves or refer patients for it.

Current research policy at the National Institute of Mental Health (NIMH) is making matters worse. Consistent with its disinterest in social sciences, NIMH now requires all mental health research grants to fit the Research Domain Criteria (RDoC) model. It asks that clinical trials be linked to neurobiological mechanisms to make them "experimental."

These decisions tend to exclude psychotherapy from NIMH research support (Goldfried, 2015).

Although some functional magnetic resonance imaging studies have shown that talking therapy can change brain connections (Linden, 2006), psychological treatment can be evaluated without links to neuroscience. We do not need biology to carry out randomized controlled trials (RCTs), the same tools that have long been applied to evaluate drug therapy, to measure the outcome of psychotherapy.

Psychiatrists who only treat psychosis and severe depression may not require a deep knowledge of psychotherapy (although it can be used as an adjunct to biological treatments). However, in common mental disorders, psychotherapy is as good as or better than psychopharmacology (Lambert, 2013). The list includes conditions for which medication is often effective (anxiety and mild to moderate depression) but for which psychotherapy produces similar results. Talking therapies can also be used in combination with drugs.

The list also includes conditions for which drugs play a marginal role and for which psychological interventions are the main form of treatment (addictions, eating disorders, and personality disorders). These conditions are common enough that every clinician should be able to ensure that patients receive appropriate treatment. Where psychiatrists lack the full range of skills required to treat these complex disorders, patients may benefit from a multidisciplinary team approach that uses individual therapy, group therapy, family therapy, and adjunctive medication. Working in a team has advantages over office practice. Addiction psychiatry often treats patients in "rehab" settings that provide individual counseling and group support (Rush 2007). Similar methods have been developed for eating disorders (Murphy, Straebler, Cooper, & Fairburn, 2010) and for personality disorders (Paris, 2015b). Thus, psychiatrists who work alone without access to a team may not always provide the most evidence-based treatment. Nonetheless, if psychiatrists are competent in psychotherapy, they can often treat these patients effectively.

CLINICAL EXPERIENCE VERSUS CLINICAL TRIALS

The reputation of psychotherapy has suffered from a tradition of being validated by clinical experience (or by the authority of gurus) rather than by systematic empirical data. Reading books or attending workshops about psychotherapy can give one an idea of what a treatment is about, but they do not tell one how well it works in the real world. That requires formal clinical trials, as well as meta-analyses to determine the generalizability of these trials.

The US Food and Drug Administration (FDA) will approve drugs using a low bar, based on only two RCTs (often paid for by the manufacturer). But it is not required to approve any method of psychotherapy. Governments do not allow pharmacological treatments to go on the market without evidence that they do no harm. But no agency exists to regulate psychological treatments. If systematic evaluation is required for the licensing of drugs, why should psychotherapies, which have equally powerful effects, be exempt?

In the absence of regulation, the practice of psychotherapy can look more like a business than an application of science. When therapists develop new methods, they cannot rely on industry or academia to spread the word. Moreover, in an already crowded marketplace, the total number of therapies endlessly increases, and many "new" methods are given a three-letter acronym to make them memorable. Often, these "named" psychotherapies are little different from existing methods. Because they are associated with the name of an expert, they can sometimes be exercises in narcissism for their creators. Also, there is money to be made by giving workshops and selling books. In a recent review of the efficacy of psychosocial treatments for mental and substance use disorders, the Institute of Medicine (2015) noted that one of the obstacles to developing evidence-based and clinically applicable treatments is the profusion of psychotherapies, each promoted by its developers.

The uniqueness of new therapies is as dubious as the marketing of "me-too" drugs. Research shows few differences in outcome between different methods of therapy. For the most part, their effects vary little from those of well-established models (Wampold, 2015). That is why it is necessary to have a single science and an integrated method of psychotherapy, using the best ideas from all sources.

In the past, hardly any psychotherapies were evidence-based. Moreover, approximately 50 years ago, many methods, with the prominent exception of behavior therapy, were variations on psychoanalysis. Aaron Beck (1986) was the first person to apply the RCT method to his own method: cognitive–behavior therapy (CBT). Today, most psychotherapies are variations on CBT, and behavior therapy has been folded into this model. The recent vogue for "third-wave" therapies, such as mindfulness or acceptance and commitment therapy (ACT), is essentially another variation, and research shows little difference in efficacy from standard

CBT (Ost, 2008). Because of its strong research base, CBT has become the favored form of psychotherapy in the eyes of both clinicians and patients.

Yet there is little evidence that CBT is superior to any other method (Baardseth et al., 2013). It is just better researched. Recently, research on other methods has been catching up. For example, there is good evidence for the efficacy of brief courses of once-weekly psychotherapy with a psychoanalytic orientation (Fonagy, 2015). But that body of research should not be interpreted as support for classical psychoanalysis or for any therapies that last for years.

Since the time of Freud, psychotherapy has been more of a craft than an applied science. Its ideas have been rooted in experience with patients. O'Donnell (1997) ironically defined clinical experience as "making the same mistakes with increasing confidence over an impressive number of years" (p. 27). In the hard world of science, experience just cannot be relied on. New ideas, no matter how promising, must be backed up with data. This is why the movement for evidence-based medicine was developed to base *all* forms of health care on solid empirical ground (Sackett, Richardson, Rosenberg, & Haynes, 1997). The same approach has been applied to clinical psychology, in which the equivalent term is "empirically supported therapies" (EST; Norcross & Goldfried, 2005).

By having agreed standards, we protect patients from quackery and provide a corrective for the tendency for therapies to multiply unnecessarily. The American Psychological Association has attempted to act as a kind of FDA for psychotherapy by publishing a list of ESTs. However, this list is insufficiently demanding, using criteria that, like those of the FDA, require only a minimum of two clinical trials.

In my view, a higher bar (both for drugs and for therapy), requiring sufficient data to conduct a meta-analysis, is called for. A better source of expert evaluation, depending on formal meta-analysis, can be found in the Cochrane reports. The Cochrane system is highly conservative, and Cochrane reports usually conclude that more evidence is needed before firm recommendations can be made. If only every clinician applied that level of caution!

Another issue is that, like drug trials, clinical trials of psychotherapies are biased when conducted by the clinician who originated the method. We all tend to see the world through the lens of our confirmation biases, leading us to misinterpret data as confirming preconceived ideas (Kahneman, 2011). This is why therapists are not the right people to evaluate the efficacy of their own treatments. They are too heavily invested in proving that their methods work.

This is also why workshops that depend on clinical examples are nearly worthless. (For this reason, I have avoided using case histories in this book to back up my arguments.) We all tend to remember our successes and forget our failures. Nor can therapists generalize from the small number of patients in their own practice to larger populations. For this reason, most books on psychotherapy lack scientific validity. It has been said that the plural of anecdote is not data. Clinical stories, no matter how well presented, never add up to real evidence. This is why all claims for psychotherapy need to be supported by systematic trials.

We now have this kind of evidence. But we did not have it until the past few decades. Interestingly, research in psychotherapy began when a widely quoted paper sharply challenged its efficacy. The British psychologist Hans Eysenck (1952) published an article titled "The Effects of Psychotherapy," suggesting that positive outcomes are no better in treated patients than in untreated patients. In his view, successful cases reflected a combination of placebo effects and naturalistic recovery. At the time, evidence-based practice was still rare, and many clinicians rejected Eysenck's critique out of hand. But the controversy that followed stimulated formal research into the outcome of psychotherapy.

During the next half century, an enormous scientific literature emerged to meet this challenge. Each year, hundreds of papers are published on the subject, and approximately every decade, findings are incorporated into a new edition of a standard text. The most recent version, the sixth edition of *Bergin and Garfield's Handbook of Psychotherapy and Behavior Change* (Lambert, 2013), summarizes the literature in approximately 1,000 pages. Let us briefly discuss what science can tell us.

WHAT SCIENCE TELLS US ABOUT PSYCHOTHERAPY

The first question everyone asks about psychotherapy is "Does it work?" The short answer is "Yes, but not always."

A vast body of evidence, supported by meta-analyses of RCTs, has shown that talking therapies are effective for a wide variety of psychological problems. All systematic reviews of the scientific evidence have come to this conclusion (Fonagy, 2015; Fonagy & Paris, 2008; Kazdin, 2008; Lambert, 2013; Lazar, 2010).

In their classic book, *The Benefits of Psychotherapy*, Smith, Glass, and Miller (1980) conducted a large-scale meta-analysis of hundreds of published studies and concluded that "psychotherapy benefits people of all ages as reliably as school educates them, medicine cures them, or business turns a profit" (p. 10). Of course, not everyone gets educated (or cured), and business does not always turn a profit. But the effect size of psychotherapy is generally approximately half a standard deviation, a moderate effect that is clinically significant. Further meta-analyses in the past few decades have not changed this verdict.

Not everyone benefits from psychotherapy, and some patients waste years in futile treatment. Nonetheless, the efficacy of psychotherapy is as good as that of most of the drugs psychiatrists prescribe.

Robyn Dawes (1994), a well-known skeptic about clinical psychology, initially doubted that psychotherapy was effective. Then, after reading the literature more carefully, and calling himself a "reformed sinner," he became convinced that it is effective. But Dawes cautioned that the effect size is neither large nor consistent, and that we do not fully understand *why* therapy works.

A parallel can be made between psychotherapy research and research on antidepressants. Neither of these treatments is a cure-all, but each plays a role in the treatment of disorders such as anxiety and depression. Their efficacy depends to a large extent on the severity of symptoms. Thus, medication is essential in severe depression, but in mild to moderate cases, psychotherapy is at least as good as drugs. The combination of both is only slightly better than either alone (Cuijpers, Sjbrandij, et al., 2009).

Most psychotherapy follows generic principles that have been called "common factors." But psychological treatment has also been adapted for managing complex clinical problems. More specific forms of therapy have been shown to be effective for patients with disorders in which drugs are not particularly helpful. Thus, psychological treatments are essential for treating substance abuse (Miller & Rollnick, 2002), eating disorders (Murphy et al., 2010), and borderline personality disorder (Paris, 2015b). Drugs are not notably useful for psychoses, but psychotherapy can sometimes add value to medication regimes (Tarrier, 2005). This is why the National Health Service in the United Kingdom has been hiring more psychologists to provide therapy to seriously ill patients, with documented increases in recovery rates (Gyani, Shafran, Layard, & Clark, 2013).

There are two complementary ways to study the effects of psychotherapy. As discussed in Chapter 5, efficacy refers to the results of RCTs. The problem with RCTs is that most patients in practice would not meet criteria for entrance into clinical trials either because they are comorbid for other diagnoses or because they are not compliant with research protocols (Zimmerman, Mattia, & Posternak, 2002). As a result, even when a therapy is shown to work, it is difficult to generalize research findings to practice (Bradley, Greene, Russ, Dutra, & Westen, 2005).

The other method of outcome assessment is research on effectiveness, the study of treatment in "naturalistic" populations (clinical settings in which no patients are excluded). However, although there is value in studying psychotherapy in the real world, effectiveness research does not use control groups. Thus, we cannot know whether patients would have gotten well with a different type of treatment, with less treatment, or with no treatment at all. Efficacy and effectiveness research on psychotherapy are complementary and offer a kind of trade-off.

HOW PSYCHOTHERAPY WORKS

The purpose of *process research* in psychotherapy is to identify mechanisms of change as therapy unfolds. The data suggest that processes common to *all* therapies are also the most important ones.

A classic book on the roots of psychotherapy (Frank & Frank, 1991) concluded, "Our survey has suggested that much, if not all, of the effectiveness of different forms of psychotherapy may be due to those features that all have in common" (p. 232). Frank and Frank argued that common factors are crucial because they inspire hope. In a way, talking therapy helps people in much the same way as does traditional religion. As they concluded, "faith may be a specific antidote for demoralization, while the mobilization of expectant trust by whatever means may be as much an etiological remedy as penicillin for pneumonia" (p. 132). Much of what can be said about how psychotherapy works is an epilogue to Frank and Frank's conclusions. However, this does not necessarily mean that specific procedures of interventions never matter.

Frank and Frank (1991) were correct in observing that psychotherapy is not just a technical procedure but also a healing relationship. The most striking confirmation comes from *comparative trials* of psychotherapy. In that kind of research, researchers randomly assign patients to different methods to determine if one is better than another. It has been consistently found that no particular form of structured treatment is more effective than any other (Wampold, 2015).

Decades ago, the American psychology professor Saul Rosenzweig (1936) reached the same conclusion. Citing Lewis Carroll's *Alice in Wonderland* (in which the dodo declares after a race that everyone has won and all shall have prizes), Rosenzweig described the absence of differences between therapies as a "dodo bird" verdict. Approximately 40 years later, Luborsky, Singer, and Luborsky (1975) found the evidence still supported this verdict. Another 40 years later, Wampold (2015) reported that the data continue to support it.

Thus, technical interventions may be less crucial than an ability to engage patients in a process. These conclusions are consistent with the idea that some therapists are better than others (Wampold, 2015). Being a good therapist may be, at least in part, a natural talent. Research shows that results do not depend on experience, gender, or training (Beutler et al., 2003). What seems to matter more is skill in getting patients engaged.

In a famous study (Strupp & Hadley, 1979), experienced therapists did no better conducting therapy than untrained university professors who had been rated by students as unusually sympathetic. These results cannot be generalized because the subjects in the study were university students in mild distress. My own research group (Propst, Paris, & Rosberger, 1994) studied patients selected for therapy in a hospital outpatient clinic. But we were also unable to find any difference in the results of brief therapy conducted by medical students, family practice residents, psychiatric residents, or staff psychiatrists. Although empathic skills can be taught (Markowitz & Milrod, 2011), some therapists are "naturals," and some are not.

The importance of talent helps explain why nonspecific factors remain the best predictors of outcome. One way to measure therapist skill is the quality of the *therapeutic alliance*—that is, the ability to work effectively with a therapist. This construct can be measured in standard scales rated by the patients. Although some patients form alliances more readily than others, a large body of research shows that even after only a few sessions of therapy, measures of the alliance allow us to predict whether treatment will be successful (Arbito & Rabellino, 2011).

Many decades ago, the American psychologist Carl Rogers (1951) conducted research to define the nature of common factors in psychotherapy. The basic elements Rogers identified were *accurate empathy, unconditional positive regard,* and *genuineness.* Thus, a good therapist understands what patients feel, has a positive attitude toward them even when they are being difficult, and is not "faking" an ability to connect with patients. However, Rogers may have put too much emphasis on qualities of the therapist and too little on the structure of treatment, which provides consistency, independent of specific interventions (Wampold, 2015).

Orlinsky, Grawe, and Parks (1994) summarized research on more than 50 different variables describing the process of psychotherapy in relation to outcome. Once again, the conclusion was that "nonspecific" factors emerged as crucial and that many of them related to a predictable structure. Thus, some of the factors that help most are a well-defined contract, a strong alliance, and a focus on current life problems and relationships. Whether therapists offer interpretations, recommend modifications of thought, or suggest ways to improve current relationships, patients do better when there is a clear plan and treatment is not allowed to drift. This is why well-structured therapies are almost always better than what researchers call "treatment as usual" (TAU)—the messy kind of practice carried out in clinics and offices.

Let us consider examples. Depression can be conceptualized not as a chemical imbalance, as biological psychiatrists would have it, but as a state of demoralization that reflects both life circumstance and underlying personality structure. This concept makes major depression a prime target for psychotherapy. In a landmark study, Elkin, Shea, Watkins, and Imber (1989) found that after excluding patients with severe symptoms (who required antidepressants), most patients got better with therapy alone, and even supportive checkups led to symptom relief. Moreover, the efficacy of two specific methods of therapy (CBT and interpersonal psychotherapy) was equal. Some studies have even suggested that "befriending" (supportive contact with unpaid but sympathetic volunteers) can be a helpful intervention for mild depression (Mead, Lester, Chew-Graham, & Gask, 2010).

Clearly, remoralization and support can be sufficient for treating patients with less severe problems. But they are unlikely to be sufficient for patients with more severe pathology, such as severe depression, chronic eating disorders, severe substance abuse, or personality disorders. These may be the cases in which specific techniques make a difference.

In my area of research, borderline personality disorder (BPD), several methods have been shown to be better than TAU (Paris, 2015b). Yet these treatments may not have effects specific to their theory or their methods. Thus, a study by McMain et al. (2009) compared dialectical behavior therapy for BPD with a procedure that applied general guidelines published by the American Psychiatric Association. The main finding, that both treatments produced identical results (with no differences at 1-year follow-up), is typical of head-to-head comparisons of structured therapies.

The failure to find differences between therapies does not imply that "anything goes." It is just that specific elements are difficult to tease out, particularly in heterogeneous clinical populations. What may be particularly difficult to measure as a specific ingredient is the work involved in getting people to function better in their work and relationships. Hope is not likely to be enough if patients lack these skills. These more subtle factors may not be present in TAU, in which the tendency is to review a patient's week and offer support without working with the patient to change his or her daily activities. In CBT, scheduling activities inside and outside the home is called *behavioral activation* (Jacobson et al., 1996). Patients with chronic disorders are either doing things wrong or are failing to try anything new, and they need a tactful explanation of how they could do better. Psychotherapies fail if they offer little more than hand-holding, as opposed to teaching the skills that patients lack. A good relationship with a therapist is necessary, but it may not be sufficient.

This is also why it is unfair to caricature psychotherapy as something any sympathetic person could do. In a book published more than 50 years ago, Schofield (1964) wondered if psychotherapy is little but "the purchase of friendship." But what Schofield missed was that understanding people in a therapy situation is an unusual skill and does not actually resemble friendship (in which people exchange confidences but do not always listen very well). In psychotherapy, the patient has the undivided attention of someone who has no axe to grind and who cares about the patient's welfare. An apocryphal story tells of a therapist who was asked how his treatment differs from friendship. His answer was, "But where would I find such a friend?"

Moreover, although it can feel good to be understood in a therapist's office, this experience may not translate into daily life in which people are much less understanding. To manage the real world, patients need to learn interpersonal skills for close relationships, friendships, and work. Skills training is a crucial element in dialectical behavior therapy, designed for patients with highly maladaptive relationships and poor emotional regulation (Linehan et al., 2015). These principles also have a broader application to psychological problems of all kinds.

WHO BENEFITS FROM PSYCHOTHERAPY?

Even the best therapists will fail when patients are not on the same page. Patient characteristics are a strong predictor of treatment outcome. Most of these predictive factors are not surprising. Patients must be cooperative, accept the framework of therapy, and be motivated to work within its structure. However, many patients have symptoms (e.g., substance abuse, eating disorders, and personality disorders) that they fail to view as problems. When treating such patients, therapists should not assume that they are ready to change their behaviors. A whole sequence of processes has to happen before they become serious about change (Prochaska, Norcross, & DiClemente, 1994). Special procedures, termed "motivational interviewing," have been developed to deal with these situations (Miller & Rollnick, 2002). Finally, patients whose functional level is higher before treatment tend to do better in treatment than those who are functioning more poorly. In this way, as a witty psychologist once stated, the rich get richer and the poor get poorer (Horwitz, 1974).

One way of assessing patient characteristics is to determine whether a personality disorder (PD) is present. Even when anxiety and depression are "comorbid," the presence of a PD strongly influences the outcome of therapy. The reason is that PD describes, by definition, long-term impairment in psychosocial functioning. Research shows that PDs can be identified in approximately half of all patients attending community clinics (Zimmerman, Chelminski, & Young, 2008). Patients with a PD do less well in therapy (Newton-Howes, Tyrer, & Johnson, 2006), and usually need specific forms of treatment tailored for their problems (Paris, 2015b). Unfortunately, PDs are often missed, probably because therapists concentrate more on symptoms they hope to relieve than on long-term patterns of interpersonal and occupational dysfunction.

Another characteristic of patients who benefit from psychotherapy is a capacity for "psychological mindedness" (McCallum & Piper, 1997). This does not refer to a Woody Allen-like tendency to prefer introspection to action. It describes the ability to observe oneself, as opposed to blaming other people or attributing distress to bodily functions. It is an essential quality for anyone who hopes to benefit from psychotherapy, but it can be taught. This capacity has been the subject of much research, including CBT methods that promote "mindfulness" (Segal, Williams, & Teasdale, 2013), as well as psychodynamic therapies that promote new thinking processes such as "mentalization" (Bateman & Fonagy, 2006).

Finally, culture affects suitability for psychotherapy. People from non-Western societies and people with limited education tend to express distress in physical rather than psychological symptoms (Kleinman, 1988). These patients may need to be offered approaches that are consistent with their cultural values and beliefs (Kirmayer, 2015). But rather like learning another language, patients can be taught how to recognize their emotions.

THE RISE AND FALL OF PSYCHOANALYSIS

The best-known psychotherapy in the 20th century was psychoanalysis, developed by Freud but modified in important ways since its early development. During a time when there was little effective treatment of any kind for mental disorders, psychoanalysis filled a niche and captured the imagination of a generation (Paris, 2005).

Very few treatments in medicine are still used 100 years after being introduced. In many ways, psychoanalysis is now a historical footnote—an idea that once had great cultural influence but did not provide enough help to patients with mental disorders. It lives on in briefer versions, such as short-term psychoanalytic therapy, which, like other brief therapies, has a respectable evidence base (Fonagy, 2015; Leichsenring & Rabung, 2011). Some of these findings have been interpreted as showing that psychoanalysis also works (Holmes, 2014). But in its original form, Freud's method has no evidence base at all.

There was a time when Freud's theories played an important, if not crucial, role in academic psychiatry (Hale, 1995). Younger psychiatrists may not remember this era. I have told this story in more detail in another book (Paris, 2005). In retrospect, I must admit the heyday of psychoanalysis was exciting in some ways. Its practitioners were often charismatic communicators, and quite a few were held in awe by psychiatry residents. They had an answer for everything and a theory that seemed to account for all human behavior. Analysts also claimed that given time and skill, they could cure the most intractable patients. This is another reason why students were attracted to them. Even today, I see the same attraction to certainty in residency programs in which psychoanalysts are active.

Some psychiatrists who later became famous for their contributions to biological research were initially attracted to psychoanalysis. Eric Kandel of Columbia University, who was awarded a 2000 Nobel Prize for his work on the neurochemistry of memory, expressed the hope that psychoanalysis could be reinvigorated by building links to neuroscience (Kandel, 1998). However, Kandel was not aware that psychotherapy had moved on since he was a student. The developer of RDoC, Thomas Insel, although he later became a leading biological psychiatrist, once felt an attraction to psychoanalytic ideas and went through a Jungian analysis while studying in San Francisco. As NIMH director, however, he was a "born-again" believer in neuroscience.

Psychoanalysis has suffered from two major problems. First, its theory of psychological development has little empirical support. Second, its method of therapy, in its original form, has never been evaluated in clinical trials. In principle, it would have been possible to recast both theory and practice into testable hypotheses, leading to revisions in both spheres. That is the way of science. But Freudian psychology was not scientific. It belonged to a prescientific era, in which clinical speculation and authority dominated many fields of medicine, including psychiatry. Because psychoanalysis told stories about the mind that could not be measured empirically and were not open to contradiction by evidence, it became a pseudoscience (Popper, 1968). Another way to understand the period of psychoanalytic hegemony is to view it as a secular religion.

After I qualified as a specialist, psychoanalysis went into a steep decline. As psychiatry became part of a movement for evidence-based medicine, the fate of Freudian ideas was sealed. Medicine treated psychoanalysis as a foreign body to be rejected.

Today, psychoanalysis survives, but only in a small niche. Many of its practitioners no longer follow Freud but, rather, prefer the more empirically based attachment model developed by John Bowlby (Cassidy & Shaver, 2016). A few researchers have promoted "neuropsychoanalysis," which claims to link Freudian theory with brain imaging (Panksepp & Solms, 2012). But you cannot support a theoretical model by cherry-picking data from neuroscience that might confirm it. The one form of psychoanalysis that has empirical support is a modified treatment: brief psychodynamic psychotherapy, which treats patients for only a few months. The results are just as good as those for CBT and other briefer therapies (Fonagy, 2015; Leichsenring, Rabung, & Leibing, 2004).

Formal psychoanalysis is the lengthiest and most expensive form of psychotherapy. Yet it has never been clinically tested beyond simple pre–post comparisons in small samples (Paris, 2005). Proponents have made attempts to show that longer periods of therapy are required for complex conditions such as personality disorders. Leichsenring and Rabung (2008) carried out a meta-analysis using studies of patients with complex psychopathology. Although these authors claimed that their results showed that longer treatments are required for these populations, their data points were few: 23 studies, of which only 11 were clinical trials with control subjects. Also, the analysis mixed findings from different conditions that might not require similar treatment. Moreover, these cohorts, drawn from specialized clinical settings, were not representative of patients seen in most psychotherapy practices. Finally, questions can be raised about whether broad conclusions can be drawn from what were rather small effect sizes. A later meta-analysis from the same authors (Leichsenring & Rabung, 2011) added a few more data points but was subject to the same limitations.

In some ways, the lack of evidence for psychoanalysis damaged the cause of psychotherapy. Biological psychiatrists who had always been suspicious of talking therapy rejoiced at the downfall of Freudian thought. Clinicians may still associate a psychological approach to treatment with the difficult-to-validate analytic model. Some older psychiatrists have made bitter comments about the nonsense they had to learn when they were residents. And it is difficult to believe how seriously these ideas were taken at the time. In his book, *Hippocrates Cried*, Michael Alan Taylor (2013) remembers this period with biting sarcasm:

> Psychological explanations for schizophrenia that placed the onus on the mother were found baseless and destructive. The notions that depression was anger inward, gastric ulcer an internalized mother's bite, and other symbolic interpretations were seen to be equally silly and subjective. (p. 15)

Because so many of its ideas invited ridicule, psychoanalysis became the author of its own decline. Yet for some time, there was no other game in town. It took time for research to develop methods of evidence-based treatment. The first such system was behavioral therapy (BT), but most psychiatrists found that approach narrow, simplistic, and inapplicable to most of the patients they saw. (As a young psychiatrist, that was precisely my view.) It took another 20 years for an alternative to be developed and tested—that is, the development of cognitive–behavioral methods. In the meantime, psychotherapy lost the support of a new generation of psychiatrists. Their motto was, "Let's get on with what we really know how to use—our expertise in pharmacology."

THE RISE OF COGNITIVE-BEHAVIORAL PSYCHOTHERAPY

A turning point came when a psychiatrist (and former psychoanalyst), Aaron Beck (1921–), devised cognitive-behavioral therapy (CBT). This approach used a comprehensive theory, backed up by a large body of empirical research, and was applicable to many conditions in clinical practice (Beck, 1986). Beck, now well into his 90s, won the Lasker Prize, the highest honor in American medicine, for this work. Unlike Freud, he conducted rigorous clinical trials to show that his methods worked—results that have been consistently confirmed (Beck, 2008). CBT eventually came to dominate the therapeutic landscape. It replaced behavior therapy, brought the mind back into treatment, linked research to practice, and created a new culture in which science was more important than rhetoric. Unlike psychoanalysis, it created a clinical culture that replaced speculation with ideas that could be empirically tested and validated using clinical trials. CBT has had an enormous impact in psychology, and it has a "toolbox" to deal with many clinical symptoms.

In contrast to psychoanalysis, CBT is commonsensical and makes no grand assumptions about the mind. As I have heard Beck say on several occasions, "There is more on the surface than meets the eye." But CBT's lack of pretension to omniscience makes it less of a magnet to young psychiatrists. CBT may have been a turning point in the history of psychotherapy, but it ran against the grain of what was happening in psychiatry and was mostly adopted by psychologists. (The Beck Institute in Pennsylvania is run by Beck's daughter Judith, who has a PhD in psychology.)

CBT does not spend years reviewing a patient's childhood experiences. Its therapists encourage patients to put the past behind them and address the present. This helps shorten the duration of treatment. Another source of strength for CBT is a clear structure and an agreed plan. Finally, a built-in feedback system encourages patients to tell therapists at the end of every session whether they feel helped.

However, we do not know whether CBT works because of its technical innovations. It may or may not be necessary to train oneself to carry out treatments that are so demanding of patients (e.g., filling out forms and keeping a diary). More likely, the secret of its success is that CBT is particularly good at tapping into the common factors that lie behind effective treatment, particularly problem-solving in the present. Contrary to common impressions, CBT is no more effective than any other method that applies these principles (Baardseth et al, 2013).

Its main competitor for extensive empirical support is interpersonal psychotherapy (IPT; Markowitz & Weissman, 2015). This method focuses on problems in intimate relationships, but its focus is on the present rather than on the past. Research on IPT, including direct comparisons to CBT (Elkin et al., 1989; Jakobsen, Hansen, Simonsen, Simonsen, & Gluud, 2012), suggests that the results of CBT do not necessarily depend on what can be found in its toolbox.

ONE PSYCHOTHERAPY, BASED IN SCIENCE

A scientific approach to psychological treatment means that there should be only *one* method—not hundreds—and that it should be called simply "psychotherapy." Its methods would be based on research findings, not on business models or therapist egos. It would use the best ideas from all current methods and be evidence-based and rooted in research findings (Norcross & Goldfried, 2005). For this to happen, psychological treatment needs to develop the same relationship to academia that drug therapy has had.

At the same time, the nature of psychotherapy research needs to change. If common factors are so powerful, we should identify them more precisely and find a way to optimize them. We also need to identify clinical problems that require more specialized methods. Even if good results are common to many methods, psychotherapy is a teachable skill. Crucially, psychotherapy needs to be focused and time-limited. To keep it brief and focused, psychological treatment requires a plan. Otherwise, it is not accountable, becoming interminable and unbearably expensive.

First and foremost, psychotherapy needs to give up the idea that treatment must be lengthy. Despite the claims of psychoanalysis and its variants, there is no evidence supporting long courses of treatment. Most therapy can be conducted effectively with a time frame of a few months. Research continues to show that extending the length of treatment brings few benefits to patients (Stiles, Barkham, & Wheeler, 2015). In fact, therapy has its strongest effects in the first few weeks (Howard, Kopta, Krause, & Orlinsky, 1986), and 3–6 months is sufficient for recovery in most patients (MacKenzie, 1996).

This is not to say that one should *never* treat patients for longer than a few months. This option may be necessary for some patients with complex mental disorders. But the evidence for lengthy therapy on a routine basis is weak. It is rare in the research literature to find comparisons of outcome in patients given shorter and longer courses of treatment. In a recent exception, Knekt et al. (2015) compared patients with anxiety and mood disorders randomly assigned to 6 months or 3 years of therapy. They found that results were equivalent on most measures and that longer treatment had a larger effect on only 2 of 13 self-report measures.

We do many things in medicine that are not firmly evidence-based. But in the absence of strong supporting data, it seems wise to set a time limit at the beginning of any psychotherapy and to think very hard (and possibly obtain a consultation from a colleague) before extending that limit. In what has been called a *stepped care* model (Bower & Gilbody, 2005), one might offer 6 months of therapy to everyone and offer a renewal only for specific reasons. It may also be useful to treat patients intermittently, providing brief modules at different points in their lives.

Moreover, we must not lose sight of cost–benefit issues. Psychotherapy is expensive, and it costs more the longer it lasts. This is the main reason it is not well insured. Time-unlimited therapy is not funded in the public sector, except in a few generous countries in northern Europe. Even if there are benefits beyond symptomatic recovery, they will apply only to a portion of the clinical population, most of whom are less severely ill. In addition, even in a public system, every long-term patient takes up resources that quickly become unavailable to patients who can benefit from shorter courses of treatment. This is why my personality disorder clinics have adopted a stepped care model.

Finally, funding extended therapy, without stronger evidence that it makes a major difference in outcome, makes little sense from a public health perspective. What does make sense, based both on cost and on scientific knowledge, is to make brief therapy the default condition. It does not matter much what theory is used or what acronym is applied. When sound general principles are applied, therapy usually works—and works rapidly.

PROBLEMS WITH PSYCHOTHERAPY RESEARCH

I have been critical of research in psychopharmacology, but some of the same problems (and some that are particular to this kind of treatment) affect psychotherapy research.

First, psychotherapy is not for everyone. Just as antidepressants help only approximately half of those for whom these drugs are prescribed, talking therapies are far from predictably successful. This is the reason why research findings are not always generalizable. As every therapist knows, some patients are too sick, insufficiently motivated, lacking in psychological mindedness, or have cultural differences that limit the benefit from this kind of intervention (Bohar & Greaves-Wade, 2013).

Second, as in psychopharmacological research, samples in research, which are usually preselected for suitability, cannot be assumed to be representative of clinical populations (Westen & Morrison, 2001). The muddle of real-world pharmacological treatment that was examined by the STAR*D project could apply equally to psychotherapy clinics.

Third, it is difficult to establish a placebo condition for clinical trials of psychotherapy. In the NIMH collaborative study of depression (Elkin et al., 1989), even sessions consisting of nothing but checkups were associated with clinical improvement. One might therefore argue that psychotherapy itself has a large component of placebo. In some ways, therapeutic skill consists of an ability to maximize these placebo effects.

Fourth, therapists who provide psychotherapy vary greatly in their abilities (Baldwin & Imel, 2013). Although evidence of a relationship between skill and outcome remains weak, it is worrying that psychotherapists do not all have the same quality of training (Weissman, Verdekui, & Gameroff, 2006).

Fifth, even if patients who benefit from psychotherapy can usually be treated briefly, we do not know how to identify populations who could do better with longer treatment. To date, the length of therapy has largely been determined by patient finances. There may be specific populations who need either a different type of therapy or some form of recovery program, but at this point we can only rely on clinical experience to identify these patients.

There are also a number of ways in which psychotherapy can go wrong in practice. First, goals are often not well defined, particularly when treatment is open-ended. This lack of structure and purpose leads to drift—an inability to critically review progress, a reluctance to terminate treatment, and a failure to consider alternatives when therapy is not going anywhere.

Second, psychotherapists have traditionally been trained to be receptive to the point of passivity and may fail to be sufficiently active and engaged with their patients. Waiting for patients to come up with their own solutions is a recipe for an irreversible stall.

Third, like biological psychiatrists, psychotherapists have a tendency to think about causation in linear terms. Whether this consists of a childhood trauma, as in psychoanalysis, or dysfunctional cognitive schema, as in CBT, theories get in the way of pragmatics and eclecticism.

Consider the common clinical scenario of post-traumatic stress disorder (PTSD), one of the few diagnoses in the *Diagnostic and Statistical Manual of Mental Disorders* (American Psychiatric Association, 2013) that assumes an etiology. However, a large body of evidence shows that traumatic experiences, by themselves, are insufficient to produce PTSD. Only a minority of those exposed become ill. Rather, predispositions, both psychological and biological, play a crucial role, and their effects are independent of severity (Breslau, Troost, Bohnert, & Luos, 2013). This is why psychotherapists who have focused on "working through" past traumas would be better advised to focus on improving current functioning. Despite a widespread perception that PTSD requires "trauma therapy" of one kind or another, a Cochrane review (Bisson, Roberts, Andrew, Cooper, & Lewis, 2013) found only weak evidence to support such methods.

WHY PSYCHIATRISTS TURNED AWAY FROM PSYCHOTHERAPY

As is the case for most professionals, treatment choices by physicians who specialize in psychiatry are influenced by a "buzz"—what their colleagues are saying and what they hear from experts. But unlike the world of psychopharmacology, industry representatives do not knock on physicians' doors offering "the latest thing" in psychotherapy. Continuing medical education focuses mostly on the latest medications, supported by speakers in the pay of industry. That is not an environment which promotes knowledge about psychological interventions and their use.

Some of the blame for the negative image of psychotherapy in medicine comes from the field itself. Long dominated by unscientific theories, psychotherapy has been perceived as failing to meet the standards of medical treatment. But psychotherapy also suffered from endless schisms and competing claims that were rarely based on science. Cognitive–behavioral therapy filled a niche and has a respectable record as an EST, but it is designed to be conducted by psychologists who are trained to do it and who find it easy to work within its framework. Also, because CBT is not a required skill in the training of most psychiatrists, physicians have been happy to let other professionals carry out this kind of treatment.

As a result, most psychotherapists today are psychologists or social workers. But their training does not always prepare them for the management of severe mental disorders. Ironically, one study (Weissman et al., 2006) found that residency in psychiatry, with all its faults, provides a better training experience in psychotherapy than graduate school in psychology or social work programs. My experience as a teacher is that many students in my department (which is relatively strong in psychotherapy) achieve a good competence in psychological treatments but fail to use it once in practice. Once graduates complete their training, the culture of contemporary psychiatry does not reinforce the development of this kind of expertise.

In this way, my profession has given up on one of its defining skills. In the past, psychiatrists prided themselves on their skills in communication. Today, many define themselves by their ability to mix psychopharmacological "cocktails." It is much easier to write prescriptions than to try to understand life stories. This situation reflects the continued split in psychiatry between two cultures—one evidence-based and hard-headed, the other poetic and fuzzy. When psychiatrists do not carry out psychotherapy (or fail to refer patients to those who do), mistreatment is possible.

However, strong scientific evidence has a way of eventually changing minds. It is quite possible that psychotherapy, despite its current decline, is due for a revival (Woolfolk, 2015). But this will not happen unless it can be demonstrated to be of real practical value in the management of difficult patients.

PSYCHOTHERAPY FOR COMMON MENTAL DISORDERS

The evidence for the efficacy of psychotherapy for common mental disorders is very strong (National Institute for Care Excellence, 2009). A recent meta-analysis (Cuijpers, Berking, et al., 2013) concluded the following:

There is no doubt that CBT is an effective treatment for adult depression, although the effects may have been over-estimated until now. CBT is also the most studied psycho-therapy for depression, and thus has the greatest weight of evidence. However, other treatments approach its overall efficacy. (p. 376)

This last point is important. Research on CBT for depression began early and is more extensive. But other methods of psy-chotherapy can produce the same results. There is strong evidence for the efficacy of short-term psychodynamic therapy in depression (Driessen, Hegelmaier, et al., 2015; Driessen, Hollon, et al., 2015). Another meta-analysis found no difference between interpersonal therapy and CBT (Jakobsen et al., 2012). The nature of depression allows many therapeutic approaches, all of which combat hopelessness, to be effective.

The findings for anxiety disorders are similar. For generalized anxiety disorder, most studies concern CBT, and its efficacy has been confirmed by a meta-analysis (Cuijpers et al., 2014). For panic disorder, CBT also has the best evidence for efficacy (Butler, Chapman, Forman, & Beck, 2015). However, many forms of psychotherapy have been found to be efficacious in the treatment of PTSD (Bradley et al., 2005).

Several other points are notable in this literature. One is that in direct comparisons of psychotherapy and pharmacotherapy for depressive and anxiety disorders, efficacy is approximately the same (Cuijpers, Berking, et al., 2013). Second, the combination of both treatments has an advantage (Cuijpers, Dekker, Hollon, & Andersson, 2009). Third, most depressed and anxious patients tend to prefer psychotherapy, if offered a choice (McHugh, Whitton, Peckham, Welge, & Ottos, 2013). In summary, talking therapies for common mental disorders stand up well to the test of clinical trials.

PSYCHOTHERAPY FOR SUBSTANCE USE, PERSONALITY DISORDERS, AND EATING DISORDERS

In other clinical domains, disorders can be more complex, more chronic, and more refractory to treatment. I repeatedly refer to substance use, personality disorders, and eating disorders because they are conditions we often see, in which medications have little role to play. Moreover, these patient populations are well known for treatment resistance and dropping out. The most effective programs use a variety of methods, generally focusing on psychosocial rehabilitation.

One of most prevalent groups of disorders seen in psychiatry is addictions. Dutra et al. (2008) summarized the research on psychotherapy for drug and alcohol use as follows:

> Effect sizes for psychosocial treatments for illicit drugs ranged from the low-moderate to high-moderate range, depending on the substance disorder and treatment under study. Given the long-term social, emotional, and cognitive impairments associated with substance use disorders, these effect sizes are noteworthy and comparable to those for other efficacious treatments in psychiatry. (p. 179)

Eating disorders present similar challenges. Wilson, Grilo, and Vitousek (2007) summarized the research literature as follows:

> Cognitive behavioral therapy is currently the treatment of choice for bulimia nervosa and binge-eating disorder, and existing evidence supports the use of a specific form of family therapy for adolescents with anorexia nervosa. Important challenges remain. Even the most effective interventions for bulimia nervosa and binge-eating disorder fail to help a substantial number of patients. (p. 199)

In personality disorders, most research concerns the borderline category, which presents frequently in clinics. Research has shown that a number of psychotherapy methods are effective for this population (Paris, 2010b). These are also patients who respond poorly to medication. I have summarized the literature as supporting a broad model of therapy rather than a specific method described by a catchy acronym (Paris, 2015c):

> There is no evidence that specific techniques make a difference in treatment outcome among BPD patients. Thus, research has not supported the idea that technical procedures or theoretical principles lead to specific therapeutic effects in BPD. Rather, patients benefit from coherent and well-structured methods that can involve different techniques and different theories. (p. 16)

Thus, although psychotherapy, by itself, is not always sufficient for management of these complex clinical problems, it has a reasonable track record in populations that are famously difficult to treat. But the populations that need treatment are huge and cannot be accommodated by the current mental health system, even if it were better funded. Specifically designed therapies are probably most useful for the sickest patients in these groups. But a broad spectrum of patients with less severe symptoms can be managed in office or outpatient practice. For example, all physicians see patients with substance use disorders, and not all of them need to go to "rehab."

A *stepped care* model, originally developed for chronic medical disorders (Davison, 2000), has been applied to chronic mental disorders (Richards, 2012). It is most suitable when a disorder is common but varies greatly in severity. The steps in stepped care involve offering simpler, more generic interventions and then applying more complex specific interventions to patients who fail to respond. In this way, one avoids the problems created by recommending specialized treatments for everyone, which leads to poor access and unmanageably long waiting lists. I have used this model as a way to manage scarce resources for the treatment of BPD (Paris, 2013). Stepped care has also been recommended for eating disorders (Wilson, Vitousek, & Loeb, 2000). The crucial point is that because psychotherapy is a resource-intensive intervention, it should be kept as brief as possible in order to be accessible.

WHY ISN'T PSYCHOTHERAPY USED MORE OFTEN?

There could be two answers to this question. First is the current zeitgeist of psychiatry, which considers psychological problems to be biological and which offers biological forms of treatment. Second is the lack of knowledge among psychiatrists concerning the strength of the evidence for the use of psychotherapy.

Medicine has little hesitation in using highly expensive interventions, such as transplants, when they can be shown to make a difference. Psychotherapy is usually more expensive than drugs in the short term but cost-effective in the long term (Gabbard, Lazar, Hornberger, & Spiegel, 1997). Psychotherapy is cost-effective because it saves money for the mental health system, mainly by reducing other medical visits. Compared to the amount of money spent on other problems in medicine, it is a bargain.

7

INTEGRATING PSYCHOTHERAPY

INTO PRACTICE

THIS CHAPTER EXAMINES HOW PSYCHOTHERAPY can be integrated into the practice of psychiatry. But this question cannot be addressed without considering how mental health services are currently delivered. Specifically, the delivery of psychiatric services may not be ideally accomplished in solo office practice but, rather, often requires multidisciplinary teams that include psychologists and social workers. This model of health care requires structures and planning that focuses on the needs of the sickest patients in the mental health system.

MENTAL HEALTH CARE SYSTEMS

Many countries, such as the United Kingdom, Australia, and Canada, have developed national mental health policies. These documents provide guidelines for the delivery of services and the human resources required to meet projected goals. The main problem with these policies is that although good intentions are always expressed, the funds required to make them work are usually lacking. (This is an example of how the stigma attached to mental illness is harmful to patients and families.)

Mental health care in the United States is different. It has what has been called a "de facto system" (Regier et al., 1993). For most potential patients, treatment is fee for service: out-of-pocket for those who can afford to pay or, for those who cannot, through insurance coverage (usually limited to a few sessions). Market forces alone determine what services are and are not available. For this reason, the model is not really a system at all. The US system is so fragmented and inconsistent that it fails to guarantee that most patients can expect to receive competent, evidence-based treatment.

The problem is not unique to psychiatry. Prior to the establishment of compulsory insurance, sick people in the United States could be threatened with bankruptcy. Even so, mental health care is poorly insured in the United States. (As I discuss later, the same problem afflicts the universal health care system in Canada.) There may be hope for change, but only in the long term.

Recently, the Institute of Medicine (IOM; England, Butler, & Gonzalez, 2015) published a report stating that approximately half of all patients in mental health facilities receive inadequate treatment, relative to standard guidelines. The authors placed emphasis on inconsistent application of evidence-based psychosocial interventions, noting that such services tend to be inadequate in the absence of multidisciplinary teams. Setting up that system costs money. Although it was too polite to say so, IOM offered a scathing criticism of American psychiatry as currently practiced. The question is whether there is enough public support to improve the system. Psychiatric illness is stigmatized, resulting in chronic underfunding and a failure to consider community needs seriously.

Mental health systems in the United Kingdom, Germany, Scandinavia, and the Netherlands are better designed, better funded, and make use of teams of multiple professional groups. Even if they do not meet all their goals, these systems make it much easier to access psychological treatment. Unlike in the United States, the health care systems in northern Europe encourage psychiatrists and psychologists to work together.

In the United Kingdom, the National Health Service (NHS) developed a program called "Improving Access to Psychological Therapies" (Clark, 2011), designed to promote broader practice by bringing more psychotherapists into mental health teams. As a result, in recent years, the NHS has hired many more clinical psychologists. The system has also been regularly evaluated since it was introduced. Not surprisingly, the main problem with the program is that demand for therapy always exceeds the supply. In a public system that pays psychiatrists and psychologists, clinicians never have to search for patients—they always have more than they can handle.

Not all public mental health systems meet the needs of the community. I know the Canadian system best. Although very different from (and in many ways superior to) the US model, health care in Canada has its own problems. Since 1970, the country has had a single-payer insurance system for universal health care paid for by taxation. Physicians are fully covered, but psychologists are not, unless they are on salary at an institution. Unless one has unusually good insurance from an employer, psychotherapy tends to be unavailable.

(In this respect, managed care in the United States is better because it treats psychiatrists and psychologists equally.)

Health service delivery in Canada is a provincial responsibility, but the federal government can set standards and put them into effect by providing or withholding transfer payments. In 2007, the federal government created the Mental Health Commission of Canada (MHCC) to establish national guidelines for the delivery of care. In a report, MHCC (2012) recommended providing access to services, expanding the role of primary care, strengthening collaboration with secondary and tertiary care, increasing availability of services in the community, setting standards for wait times, and increasing access to evidence-based psychotherapies—all of which IOM has recommended for the United States.

This strategy clearly means that psychiatrists should work as consultants to primary care services and devote most of their direct clinical time to the sickest patients. The model in which psychiatrists support less specialized caregivers, thereby reaching a wider population, is called *shared care* (Kates et al., 2006).

These recommendations are the same as those made three decades ago by the Canadian psychiatrist Heinz Lehmann (1986). Lehmann, one of my most influential teachers, suggested that psychiatrists should not necessarily treat common mental disorders in office practice. Instead, they could take on a new role, defined by a focus on acute care, the care of the chronically mentally ill, and conducting outreach through consultation. Lehmann's view was that because psychotherapy does not require a medical degree, these services can be provided by other health professionals. The main problem was that Lehmann failed to consider financial barriers to treatment outside a public system.

Nonetheless, the model has been applied, at least partially, in many provinces of Canada, particularly in university teaching hospitals.

In Canada, there is good access to acute care, but there can be significant waiting lists for long-term treatment and rehabilitation programs. The main problem for the mental health system is that psychologists, who are best placed do this work, are almost entirely unfunded. When a psychiatrist provides psychotherapy, it is fully insured by the government, with minimal to no restrictions on frequency of sessions or length of treatment. But as discussed previously, most psychiatrists currently offer little psychotherapy, and those who do are flooded with demands they cannot meet.

The reason for not insuring psychologists in Canada is similar to that for limiting coverage for psychotherapy under US managed care. Psychological treatment has a reputation for being interminable and for being provided to the "worried well." The Canadian system could have addressed these objections by limiting the number of sessions to 20 per year, a length supported by evidence (MacKenzie, 1996). Also, it could have taken into account evidence that brief courses of psychotherapy reduce total medical costs (Gabbard, Lazar, Hornberger, & Spiegel, 1997; Roth & Fonagy, 2005). However, provincial health insurance has never covered any of the services of psychologists working outside hospitals, in contrast to universal access in some health care systems in Europe. Thus, Canadian patients have no better access to evidence-based psychotherapy than their American neighbors. An additional problem is that there is no assurance of quality in psychotherapy, even when patients pay for it. (However, this is not different from the absence of serious oversight of any of the practices of physicians.)

PSYCHIATRISTS AND MENTAL HEALTH TEAMS

Insuring physicians is insufficient to establish an accessible and effective mental health system. Effective care requires multidisciplinary teams, particularly the inclusion of clinical psychologists. Let us examine how multidisciplinary mental health teams would operate. Psychiatrists would be primarily responsible for making diagnoses and providing psychopharmacological interventions. Psychologists and social workers would do most of the psychotherapy, particularly for patients with common mental disorders. Psychiatrists, however, would be trained to conduct therapy themselves on the most complex cases.

Contrast this model to the current system in which psychiatrists, often working alone, can only use the tools they know best—that is, prescriptions. When physicians believe that drugs are the one and only form of treatment they have to offer, these agents tend to be offered to almost every patient.

In some areas of the United States, there is a shortage of physicians to write prescriptions for patients with common mental disorders. (But given the empirical evidence shedding doubt on the efficacy of antidepressants in larger populations, one wonders whether the shortage is good or bad.) There are approximately 45,000 psychiatrists in the United States, insufficient by themselves (especially considering geographical maldistribution) to provide services to a population of 350 million people. However, there are approximately 200,000 primary care physicians in the United States, and they have long been writing more prescriptions for antidepressants than psychiatrists (Pincus et al., 1998).

Primary caregivers could carry even more of the load if they had ready access to psychiatric consultation.

I have often heard psychiatrists state that depressed patients are undertreated. This conclusion has led to the idea that we need to promote psychiatric diagnoses and antidepressant prescriptions. Some advocates have set up shop in malls, administering screening questionnaires to passers-by. Although surveys show that a large number of people with depressed and anxious symptoms are not receiving any treatment (Kessler et al., 2005), it does not necessarily follow that most of them need to be on medication.

The belief that drugs are necessary for common mental disorders is so strong that it has been suggested that clinical psychologists with a doctoral degree should be allowed to prescribe after receiving additional training (American Psychological Association, 2011). These prescribing privileges are currently recognized in three US states (Illinois, New Mexico, and Louisiana), as well as in the US military. There are no data on the outcome of this policy, but I doubt that it is necessary. If patients require antidepressants, other alternatives could meet these needs, including better training and support for primary care physicians, as well as multidisciplinary mental health teams in which psychologists and psychiatrists work closely together. The other profession that could fill the gap, particularly in regions where physician supply is short, is the nurse practitioner. Also, it is possible that many untreated people in the community could be more effectively treated with psychotherapy.

I am very concerned that if psychologists obtain privileges to treat patients with drugs, they will overprescribe at the same rate that we now see among physicians. The same pressures would lead to much the same outcome. (Even if they did not want to give out drugs, their patients would insist on a prescription.) It is strange to be concerned that patients are not getting the benefit of drugs when we know that antidepressants are not always better than placebo (Kirsch et al., 2008) and when between 10% and 15% of the population is already taking these agents (Kantor, Rehm, Haas, Chan, & Giovannucci, 2015; Pratt et al., 2011). Advocates of expanding prescribing privileges to psychologists do not consider that overprescription is as great a danger as underprescription (or even a greater danger). If psychologists had this privilege, the rate of antidepressant use might easily increase up to 25%. Even worse, clinical psychologists, like psychiatrists, would be driven by market forces to move away from practicing psychotherapy. (That is why many psychologists who actively practice therapy are against these proposals.)

Instead of turning every mental health professional into a biological psychiatrist, it would make more sense to create a team to which members contribute their unique skills. In this model, psychiatrists would devote more of their time to providing consultation and support to primary care physicians and psychologists, thereby making the best use of their unique expertise. Psychiatrists could still provide direct treatment, but they could concentrate on the sickest patients—the cases that primary care providers (and many psychologists) tend to find difficult (e.g., chronically suicidal patients).

In this model, psychiatrists would retain a key role in teams that provide comprehensive care to patients with severe mental illness without, as tends to happen in community mental health centers, limiting themselves to conducting med checks on patients followed by other professionals. Another problem with a med-check practice is that psychiatrists lose any skills they may have once had in psychotherapy, and they cannot contribute this knowledge to team discussions.

Links between specialized mental health care and primary care are important for this model. The concept of *shared care* is beginning to be used in Canada, although it has not yet been applied consistently. Psychiatrists are encouraged to spend more time on consultation (by receiving higher fees than for direct care). However, these incentives have been insufficient to keep many psychiatrists, particularly those who work in their own offices, from seeing only patients with whom they feel comfortable (Paris, Goldbloom, & Kurdyak, 2015). Thus, although the intentions of the Canadian system are good, its results are far from optimal. There is also a serious shortage of primary care physicians because medical graduates prefer to pursue lucrative specialty practices.

Nonetheless, the situation is better than it used to be. I lived through the transition from a private to a public system in Canada in 1970. Prior to the institution of universal health insurance, the practice of psychiatry was in every way private, not greatly different from the current model in the United States. After the establishment of publically funded medicine, patients with severe psychopathology were more likely to be seen by psychiatrists (Sareen, Cox, Afifi, Yu, & Stein, 2005). There was no longer any need for psychiatrists to find wealthy people or families who could pay their fees. (And because the wealthy no longer had privileged access to services, many had to access the public system through hospital clinics.) The Canadian system is inadequately funded, but in terms of accessibility, it is equally fair (or unfair) to everyone. The system has no lack of problems, but few of my colleagues would prefer to work in the United States.

INCORPORATING PSYCHOTHERAPY INTO PSYCHIATRIC PRACTICE

Mojtabai and Olfson (2008) reported a striking decline over time in the number of psychiatrists who provide psychotherapy to all patients, from 19.1% in 1996–1997 to 10.8% in 2004–2005. The percentage of visits involving psychotherapy also declined, from 44.4% in 1996–1997 to 28.9% in 2004–2005. Although nearly 60% of psychiatrists reported providing psychotherapy to at least some of their patients, the quality of these interventions is not known.

These data are now more than 10 years old, and I suspect the situation is getting worse. Psychotherapy was defined in the survey as sessions lasting at least 30 minutes. Taking time to listen to patients is a major improvement over a med check, and no one has carried out research to determine what the proper length of a session should be. However, it is difficult to determine whether psychiatrists are providing evidence-based psychotherapy. Also, it is not known if psychiatrists report their activities accurately in surveys.

Family physicians could, with suitable training, also carry out psychotherapy. Time constraints are often given as a reason why this is impractical in primary care settings. However, more than half a century ago, Castelnuevo-Tedesco (1965) suggested a 20-minute "hour," using an active and focused approach for current life problems that could fit into the schedule of a primary care physician. Relatively recently, a group of psychologists trained in cognitive–behavioral therapy (CBT) made a similar suggestion, calling their 15- to 20-minute segments "high-yield CBT" (Wright, Sudak,

Turkington, & Thase, 2010). However, the authors noted that it would be difficult to carry out effective work in 15 minutes unless one had previous experience delivering therapy in a standard 45- to 50-minute session.

Every psychiatry residency program is required to promote competency in psychotherapy. But the quality of training varies greatly. There is less oversight of residency in the United States than in Canada. Even so, American psychiatry residents receive, on average, better training in psychological treatment than psychologists or social workers (Weissman, Verdekui, & Gameroff, 2006). The problem is that they do not use these skills once residency is over and, therefore, lose them. Psychiatrists may say they have no time to do psychotherapy. More accurately, they may not feel competent to carry it out. Given these constraints, it may well be unrealistic to expect most psychiatrists to give a major place to psychotherapy in their practice anytime soon.

Access is a matter of not only cost but also availability of resources. There will never be enough psychiatrists to meet the needs of most patients with common mental disorders. That is why psychiatry can do more for this population by being consultants to primary care physicians, psychologists, and social workers.

Even so, psychiatrists who have skills in psychotherapy could provide better service to all their patients. If their only experience was during residency, and their memory about these methods is vague, it will be difficult to collaborate with other professionals who routinely practice therapy. That is why I recommend that psychiatrists in teams take a few patients in regular therapy, just to stay involved in it. These patients should preferably have complex problems that require an experienced clinician. These cohorts may also benefit from treatment that is not divided between two or more professionals.

SPLIT TREATMENT

Split treatment describes a model in which different professionals provide different types of treatment to the same patient. From a practical standpoint, given a limited number of psychiatrists, and the lack of training in psychotherapy among non-psychiatric physicians, split treatment is inevitable for most patients. But under certain conditions, the split can be problematic.

In 2001, Gabbard and Kay argued that split treatment reinforces an artificial separation of the psychosocial and biological domains in psychiatry. They noted that although research often supports combined treatment for conditions such as depression, it is not known whether patients benefit from having services provided by different professionals or whether integrated treatment remains best. Dewan (1999) concluded that split treatment has few advantages in cost-effectiveness. But given the number of mental health professionals relative to the demand for therapy, split treatments for most patients are probably inevitable. Psychiatrists who treat only patients who are economically privileged may not be in tune with the larger problems of mental health care delivery.

There has been little research in this area. Thus, I can only raise concerns derived from my own experience. One is that split treatment can lead to more prescriptions than are necessary. A psychologist who is working with a psychiatrist, and who is anxious about a patient, may insist that drugs be given. Thus, a prescription is very likely to be written, and if a patient has not responded to one already given, the result is a raised dose or another medication. In this way, split treatment can be an illusory source of comfort for a psychotherapist. When things are difficult or not going well, therapists fall back on the hope that medication will break the cycle. But in a team setting, they have the option of considering how to improve psychological treatment. The availability of a wider range of options for difficult patients is what makes it interesting to be a psychiatrist.

The argument is often made that because psychiatrists are physicians, they should concentrate on the skills they know and understand best, leaving psychotherapy to other professionals. This may be reasonable for psychiatrists who work in hospitals and who spend their time treating patients with psychoses, melancholic depression, and dementia. However, this view is badly mistaken with regard to the management of patients with common mental disorders.

First, psychiatrists do not necessarily refer patients who are suitable for psychotherapy to other professionals. I have discussed limited insurance as one reason. But for many psychiatrists, the option does not even come to mind. They believe in their medications and almost always prescribe them. I work in an outpatient setting and have read thousands of consultations from my colleagues. They *always* suggest drugs, and they often suggest several drugs. That is why so many patients with depression, anxiety, or personality disorder are on two antidepressants, one antipsychotic, a sleeping pill, and may also be prescribed stimulants. I believe that I am one of very few who will recommend stopping unnecessary drugs and considering a referral for psychotherapy. This behavior by psychiatrists may only be understandable as having only a hammer and seeing only nails. Moreover, psychiatrists who never do psychotherapy are particularly likely to depend entirely on pharmacology.

Second, the splitting of treatment between psychologists and psychiatrists is not optimal for patients. Two busy clinicians do not always talk to each other. When symptoms do not remit, the psychiatrist will probably prescribe more aggressively. When psychotherapy is not going well, a psychologist may request a change in medication. Missing from this picture is the value of a single clinician, skilled in both approaches, who can make more informed decisions.

A STEPPED CARE MODEL

Another way to make service delivery is to adopt a stepped care model. This strategy would offer less intensive treatment as a first step, reserving resource-intensive rehabilitation methods as a second step for those who do not improve (Bower & Gilbody, 2005). The greatest benefit of this approach is that it does not waste precious resources on patients who can get better with less intensive and briefer interventions. Stepped care triages cases in a way that tends to eliminate waiting lists, opening up more places for acute care. Finally, stepped care could be more accountable.

This principle is particularly relevant to the use of psychotherapy. Simply continuing treatments when they are not working is a road to futility. Clinicians also have to accept that not every patient they see will emerge fully remitted or "cured." Also, many patients continue to improve after the end of treatment. The failure to take long-term prognosis into account is an example of what Cohen and Cohen (1984) called the "clinician's illusion"—that is, a misperception based on the fact that recovered patients tend to stop coming for treatment, whereas unrecovered patients continue to ask for treatment.

In my own clinical work, I apply these principles to the management of patients with BPD (Paris, 2013). Many in this population can be treated briefly, providing a boost to a natural process of recovery. Expensive and time-intensive interventions can be reserved for the most chronic patients. Applying this model would reduce costs and make brief therapy more accessible to patients who are known to benefit from it.

Triage is the central principle of stepped care. Its advantage is that this is a model of care that husbands scarce resources. Most patients in the mental health system will remit to the point where they can either be fully discharged or be followed in primary care. This is even true of schizophrenia, which rarely continues to present acute symptoms by middle age (Harding, Brooks, Ashikaga, Strauss, & Brier, 1987).

Finally, this model allows for a more effective use of psychotherapeutic skills for both acutely ill and chronically ill patients. Instead of being a nonspecific support, psychotherapy can become one of a large variety of tools that put patients on a trajectory to recovery.

CONTROLLING THE COST OF PSYCHOTHERAPY

In medicine, expensive treatments for patients may be insurable if costs are justified by empirical data for efficacy. When complex interventions are evidence-based, as is the case in transplantation medicine, cardiac surgery, or oncology, there may be no political resistance to obtaining public funds for expensive treatments. Is there equally strong data that could justify the use of psychotherapy in the practice of psychiatry? The answer is yes, but only for brief therapy. This is a much less costly option than procedures that, due to public demand, are insured despite their expense.

There are many reasons why psychotherapy is poorly insured, including the stigma of mental illness and the stubborn belief that talking cannot help deeply troubled people. But psychotherapy has brought some of these negative perceptions on itself. There is no definite endpoint to therapy, and patients who can afford to pay for it are reluctant to give it up. Moreover, therapists whose income depends on filling a practice find reasons to continue treatment for months or years.

Given that long-term treatment is expensive and has a weak evidence base, insuring it without a limit on the number of sessions of psychotherapy would be irresponsible. One of the most consistent findings in the large empirical literature on psychotherapy outcome is that when psychotherapy works, it takes effect rapidly and can generally be limited to a duration of 6 months (Howard, Kopta, Krause, & Orlinsky, 1986; MacKenzie, 1996). Also, open-ended treatment contracts at the beginning of treatment are clinically regressive because they fail to encourage activation and coping. Moreover, because almost all the evidence for the efficacy of psychotherapy is based on treatments lasting 6 months or less, psychological treatment in the mental health system should be brief and targeted. There may still be a minority of patients who need more than 6 months of therapy. However, this option should not be used unless there is good evidence for doing so, as is done in rehabilitation programs for the most chronic patients (Rossler, 2006).

INTEGRATING PSYCHOTHERAPY INTO PRACTICE

Psychotherapy is an evidence-based treatment for a wide variety of disorders. It should therefore be an important tool for psychiatrists. But that does not mean that they always need to provide this treatment on their own. The demand is much too great and time much too limited.

However, psychiatrists should know how to provide brief therapy for mental disorders. They should also be trained to carry out psychological interventions for complex conditions such as substance abuse, eating disorders, and personality disorders. In addition, they should be prepared to work in teams with other professionals and to refer less complex patients to psychologists (or other nonmedical professionals). Nonmedical therapists can be supported by providing consultation, guidance, and support in crises, and medication can be prescribed when clearly indicated.

The solo office practice of psychiatry is becoming an anachronism. A biopsychosocial model of treatment is best carried out in a team setting (Paris et al., 2015). Increasingly more often, psychiatrists work as consultants in multidisciplinary teams that offer care to a wide clinical population. But the sickest patients should always be the first priority for highly trained medical specialists. Their skills are needed to provide direct care, including both medication and psychotherapy, to the most severely ill patients.

This model makes the best use of a psychiatrist's unique skills while husbanding scarce resources. But it requires that psychiatrists know how to conduct psychotherapy or, at the very least, when to refer to others for psychological treatment.

EPILOGUE

Psychiatry and Humanism

AS THE SCIENCE BEHIND PSYCHIATRY has progressed, it has lost much of its humanism. In some ways, humanism is like motherhood. Hardly anyone admits being against it, even if their actions speak otherwise. And humanism is what attracted so many medical graduates in my generation to go into psychiatry. We wanted to see every patient as a person, not as a mix of chemicals. Yes, some mental disorders are very like medical illnesses, and they can be understood in the same way. But most arise from a patient's life story and unique history. This is precisely why psychiatry needs to regain its humanistic traditions.

A good deal has been written about the importance of seeing a patient as a person in medicine (Gould & Lipkin, 1999). Hard-headed biological psychiatrists may dismiss this view of the doctor–patient relationship as irrelevant or sentimental. They prefer to get on with "real" medicine. Nonetheless, as we have seen in psychotherapy research, an empathic relationship has great healing potential. Even when drugs are indicated, there is no reason to practice entirely on the basis of med checks. Moreover, results are likely to be better when patients feel respected and understood.

I have suggested some of the things that are wrong with psychiatry. But there are also many things that are right. The specialty is making progress in understanding and treating disorders of the mind that present some of the most difficult problems in medicine. During the past few decades, it has been a privilege to practice psychiatry.

But to be a psychiatrist these days, you need a thick skin. The field is under constant attack by a hostile "antipsychiatry" movement that is ignorant about both mind and brain. At the same time, our medical colleagues do not understand what we do. Many retain a stigmatic view of psychopathology— unless, of course, they or their families have been affected by mental illness. Some of our patients are disappointed in what we can do for them—and they may be right in the sense that we often help but rarely cure.

Throughout the years since I was a student, psychiatry and medicine have become much more scientific. This has led to a change in the climate of training. Residents no longer take everything their teachers say as gospel. They are taught, in journal clubs and in evidence-based medicine seminars, to take a skeptical view of how much we know and whether our treatments actually work. Sometimes the complexity of the field is too daunting, tempting trainees to accept simplistic views promoted by narrow-minded teachers. But most of us agree that the quality of our trainees is much higher than it was in the past.

Young psychiatrists may be knowledgeable, but only some know how to take the time to sit with troubled patients, and only some have the imagination and the acumen to empathize with their experiences. Psychotherapy, once overutilized in the treatment of mental disorders, is now seriously underutilized.

Many forces have combined to change psychiatry in the way described in this book. First and foremost is a quest for legitimacy, based on neuroscience. Second is the powerful influence of the pharmaceutical industry. Third is the split between psychiatry and psychology, leading to a failure to acknowledge a large body of evidence about treatment. Fourth is the way psychiatrists are paid. Fifth is the enormous and constantly increasing demand for mental health services.

This book has proposed ways in which the situation could change. First, psychiatry needs to return to a biopsychosocial model, and its practitioners need to think in terms of interactions rather than linear relationships. Second, we need to end our troubled marriage to the pharmaceutical industry with a separation. Third, psychiatrists need to be taught more about psychology and psychotherapy. Fourth, psychiatrists should not be paid in a fee-for-service model that discourages spending time with patients. Fifth, we need to move out of offices and work in teams, sharing care with other professionals, particularly clinical psychologists.

All this is easier said than done. My voice is not the only one; my colleague Allen Frances (2013) has taken a very similar view. But in the end, change has to come from consumers—patients and their families. When psychiatry was "brainless," the National Association for the Mentally Ill played an important role in fighting against the blaming of families and for reduced stigma and increased access to treatment. What needs to happen now is different—a recognition that patients are people and that mental disorders are more than brain disorders. Such a change may take time.

And none of this is likely to happen until we adopt a better model of health service delivery.

For all these reasons, psychotherapy in an age of neuro-science needs advocacy. The cause may not have as strong a voice as the latest drug, but it demands to be heard.

REFERENCES

American Psychiatric Association. (1980). *Diagnostic and statistical manual of mental disorders* (3rd ed.). Washington, DC: Author.

American Psychiatric Association. (2010). *Practice guideline for the treatment of major depressive disorder.* Retrieved from https://psychiatryonline.org/pb/assets/raw/sitewide/practice_guidelines/guidelines/mdd.pdf

American Psychiatric Association. (2013). *Diagnostic and statistical manual of mental disorders* (5th ed.). Arlington, VA: American Psychiatric Publishing.

American Psychiatric Association. (2015). Five things physicians and patients should question. *Choosing Wisely.* Retrieved from http://www.choosingwisely.org/societies/american-psychiatric-association

American Psychological Association. (2011). Practice guidelines regarding psychologists' involvement in pharmacological issues. *American Psychologist, 66,* 835–849.

Anderson, I. M. (2000). Selective serotonin reuptake inhibitors versus tricyclic antidepressants: A meta-analysis of efficacy and tolerability. *Journal of Affective Disorders, 58,* 19–36.

Andreasen, N. C. (2001). *Brave new brain: Conquering mental illness in the era of the genome.* New York, NY: Oxford University Press.

Arbito, R. B., & Rabellino, D. (2011). Therapeutic alliance and outcome of psychotherapy: Historical excursus, measurements, and prospects for research. *Frontiers in Psychology, 2,* 270–279.

Avorn, J. (2004). *Powerful medicines: The benefits, risks, and costs of prescription drugs.* New York, NY: Knopf.

Baardseth, T. P., Goldberg, S. B., Pace, B. T., Wislocki, A. P., Frost, N. D., Siddiqui, J. R., . . . Wampold, B. E. (2013). Cognitive-behavioral therapy versus other therapies: Redux. *Clinical Psychology Review 33,* 395–405.

Baker, D. B. (2011). *The Oxford handbook of the history of psychology: Global perspectives.* New York, NY: Oxford University Press.

Baldessarini, R. J. (2014). The impact of psychopharmacology on contemporary Psychiatry. *Canadian Journal of Psychiatry, 59,* 401–405.

Baldwin, S. A., & Imel, Z. E. (2013). Therapist effects: Findings and methods. In M. Lambert (Ed.), *Handbook of psychotherapy and behavior change* (pp. 258–297). New York, NY: Wiley.

Barlow, D. (2010). Negative effects from psychotherapy: A perspective. *American Psychologist, 65,* 13–20.

Bateman, A., & Fonagy, P. (2006). *Mentalization based treatment: A practical guide.* New York, NY: Wiley.

Bedau, M. A., & Humphreys, P. (Eds.). (2008). *Emergence: Contemporary readings in philosophy and science.* Cambridge, MA: MIT Press.

Beck, A. T. (1986). *Cognitive therapy and the emotional disorders.* New York, NY: Basic Books.

Beck, A. T. (2008). The evolution of the cognitive model of depression and its neurobiological correlates. *American Journal of Psychiatry, 165,* 969–977.

Beck, A. T., & Haigh, E. (2014). Advances in cognitive theory and therapy: The generic cognitive model. *Annual Review of Clinical Psychology, 10,* 1–24.

Belsky, J., & Pluess, M. (2009). Beyond diathesis stress: Differential susceptibility to environmental influences. *Psychological Bulletin, 35,* 885–908.

Bentall, R. P. (2003). *Madness explained: Psychosis and human nature.* London, UK: Penguin.

Bentall, R. P. (2010). *Doctoring the mind.* New York, NY: Penguin.

Beutler, L. E., Malik, M., Alimohamed, S., Harwood, M., Talchi, H., Noble, S., & Wong, E. (2003): Therapist variables. In M. J. Lambert (Ed.), *Bergin and Garfield's Handbook of Psychotherapy and Behavior Change* (pp. 227–230). New York, Wiley.

Bisson, J. I., Roberts, N., Andrew, M., Cooper, R., & Lewis, C. (2013, December 13). Psychological therapies for chronic post-traumatic stress disorder (PTSD) in adults. *Cochrane Database of Systematic Reviews* (12), CD003388.

Bohart, A. C., & Greaves-Wade, A. (2013): The Client in Psychotherapy. In M. Lambert (Ed.), *Handbook of Psychotherapy and Behavior Change* (pp. 219–225). New York Wiley.

Borrell-Carrio, F., Suchman, A. L., & Epstein, R. M. (2004). The biopsychosocial model 25 years later: Principles, practice, and scientific inquiry. *Annals of Family Medicine, 2,* 576–582.

Bower, P., & Gilbody, S. (2005). Stepped care in psychological therapies: Access, effectiveness and efficiency. *British Journal of Psychiatry, 186,* 11–17.

Bradley, R., Greene, J., Russ, E., Dutra, L., & Westen, D. (2005). A multidimensional meta-analysis of psychotherapy for PTSD. *American Journal of Psychiatry, 162,* 214–277.

Breslau, N., Chilcoat, H., Kessler, R. C., & Davis, G. C. (1999). Previous exposure to trauma and PTSD effects of subsequent trauma: Results from the Detroit Area Survey of Trauma. *American Journal of Psychiatry, 56,* 902–907.

Breslau, N., Troost, J. P., Bohnert, K., & Luos, Z. (2013). Influence of predispositions on post-traumatic stress disorder: Does it vary by trauma severity? *Psychological Medicine, 43,* 381–390.

Burmeister, M., McInns, M. G., & Zollner, S. (2008). Psychiatric genetics—Progress amid controversy. *Nature Reviews Genetics, 9,* 527–540.

Burton, R. A. (2014). *A skeptic's guide to the mind: What neuroscience can and cannot tell us about ourselves.* New York, NY: St. Martin's Press.

Butler, A. C., Chapman, J. E., Forman, E. M., & Beck, A. T. (2015). The empirical status of cognitive–behavioral therapy: A review of meta-analyses. *Clinical Psychology Review, 26,* 17–31.

Cacioppo, J. T., Cacioppo, S., Dulawa, S., & Palmer, A. A. (2014). Social neuroscience and its potential contribution to psychiatry. *World Psychiatry, 13,* 131–139.

Cannon, T. D., & Keller, M. C. (2006). Endophenotypes in the genetic analyses of mental disorders. *Annual Review of Clinical Psychology, 2,* 267–290.

Cantor-Graae, E., & Selten, J. P. (2005). Schizophrenia and migration: A meta-analysis and review. *American Journal of Psychiatry, 162,* 12–24.

Carlat, D. (2010). *Unhinged: The trouble with psychiatry—A doctor's revelations about a profession in crisis.* New York, NY: Simon & Schuster.

Carroll, B. (2010). Antipsychotic drugs for depression? *American Journal of Psychiatry, 167,* 216.

Carroll, B. (2015). Clinical science and biomarkers: Against RDoC. *Acta Psychatrica Scandinavica, 132,* 423–424.

Carvalho, A. F., Cavalcante, J. L., Castelo, S., & Lima, M. (2007). Augmentation strategies for treatment-resistant depression: A literature review. *Journal of Clinical Pharmacy and Therapeutics, 32,* 415–428.

Caspi, A., McClay, J., Moffitt, T. E., Mill, J., Martin, J., & Craig, I. W. (2002). Role of genotype in the cycle of violence in maltreated children. *Science, 297,* 851–854.

Caspi, A., Sugden, K., Moffitt, T. E., Taylor, A., Craig, I. W., & Harrington, H. (2003). Influence of life stress on depression: Moderation by a polymorphism in the 5-HTT gene. *Science, 301,* 386–389.

Cassidy, J., & Shaver, P. R. (2016). *Handbook of attachment: Theory, research, and clinical applications* (3rd ed.). New York, NY: Guilford.

Castelnuevo-Tedesco, P. (1965). *The Twenty-Minute Hour: A Guide to Brief Psychotherapy for the Physician.* Boston, Little Brown.

Chalmers, D. J. (1996). *The conscious mind: In search of a fundamental theory.* New York, NY: Oxford University Press.

Chen, J., Gao, K., & Kemp, D. E. (2011). Second-generation antipsychotics in major depressive disorder: Update and clinical perspective. *Current Opinion in Psychiatry, 24,* 10–17.

Churchland, P. (1986). *Neurophilosophy: Toward a unified science of the mind–brain.* Cambridge, MA: MIT Press.

Ciccheti, D., & Rogosch, F. (1996). Equifinality and multifinality in developmental psychopathology. *Development and Psychopathology, 8,* 597–600.

Cipriani, A., Furukawa, T. A., Salanti, G., Geddes, J. R., Higgins, J. P. T., Churchill, R., ... Barbui, C. (2009). Comparative efficacy and acceptability of 12 new-generation antidepressants: A multiple-treatments meta-analysis. *Lancet, 373,* 746–758.

Cipriani, A., Pretty, H., Hawton, K., & Geddes, J. R. (2005). Lithium in the prevention of suicidal behavior and all-cause mortality in patients with mood disorders: A systematic review of randomized trials. *American Journal of Psychiatry, 162,* 1805–1819.

Clark, D. M. (2011). Implementing NICE guidelines for the psychological treatment of depression and anxiety disorders: The IAPT experience. *International Review of Psychiatry, 23,* 375–384.

Cohen, P., & Cohen, J. (1984). The clinicians' illusion. *Archives of General Psychiatry, 41,* 1178–1182.

Corrigan, P. W. (Ed.). (2005). *On the stigma of mental illness: Practical strategies for research and social change.* Washington, DC: American Psychological Association.

Coyle, J. T. (2005). Julius Axelrod (1912–2004). *Molecular Psychiatry, 10,* 225–226.

Coyle, J. T. (2006). Glutamate and schizophrenia: Beyond the dopamine hypothesis. *Cellular and Molecular Neurobiology, 26,* 365–384.

Crick, F. (1995). *The astonishing hypothesis: The scientific search for the soul.* New York, NY: Scribner.

Crossley, N. A., Scott, J., Ellison-Wright, I., & Mechelli, A. (2015). Neuroimaging distinction between neurological and psychiatric disorders. *British Journal of Psychiatry, 207,* 429–434.

Cuijpers, P., Berking, M., Andersson, G., Quigley, L., Kleiboer, A., & Dobson, K. S. (2013). A meta-analysis of cognitive–behavioural therapy for adult depression, alone and in comparison with other treatments. *Canadian Journal of Psychiatry, 58,* 376–385.

Cuijpers, P., Dekker, J., Hollon, S. D., & Andersson, G. (2009). Adding psychotherapy to pharmacotherapy in the treatment of depressive disorders in adults: A meta-analysis. *Journal of Clinical Psychiatry, 70,* 1219–1229.

Cuijpers, P., Sjbrandij, M., Koole, S., Andersson, G., Berking, M., & Reynolds, C. F. (2013), The efficacy of psychotherapy and pharmacotherapy in treating depressive and anxiety disorders: A meta-analysis of direct comparisons. *World Psychiatry, 12,* 137–148.

Cuijpers, P., Sjbrandij, M., Koole, S., Huibers, M., Berking, M, & Andersson, G. (2014). A psychological treatment of generalized anxiety disorder: A meta-analysis. *Clinical Psychology Review, 34,* 130–140.

Cuthbert, B. N. (2014). The RDoC framework: Facilitating transition from ICD/DSM to dimensional approaches that integrate neuroscience and psychopathology. *World Psychiatry, 13,* 28–35.

Cuthbert, B. N., & Insel, T. R. (2013). Toward the future of psychiatric diagnosis: The seven pillars of RDoC. *BMC Medicine, 11,* 126.

Cuthbert, B. N., & Kozak, M. J. (2013). Constructing constructs for psychopathology: The NIMH Research Domain Criteria. *Journal of Abnormal Psychology, 122,* 928–937.

Davison, G. C. (2000). Stepped care: Doing more with less? *Journal of Consulting and Clinical Psychology 68,* 580–585.

Dawes, R. M. (1994). *House of cards: Psychology and psychotherapy built on myth.* New York, NY: Free Press.

De Simoni, M. G., DeLuigi, A., Clavenna, A., & Manfridi, A. (1992). In vivo studies on the enhancement of serotonin reuptake by tianeptine. *Brain Research, 574,* 93–97.

Deacon, T. (2011). *Incomplete nature: How mind emerged from matter.* New York, NY: Norton.

Decker, H. S. (2013). *The making of DSM-III: A diagnostic manual's conquest of American psychiatry.* New York, NY: Oxford University Press.

Deisseroth, K. (2011). Optogenetics. *Nature Methods, 8,* 26–29.

Dennett, D. (1996). *Darwin's dangerous idea: Evolution and the meanings of life.* New York, NY: Touchstone.

Dewan, M. (1999). Are psychiatrists cost-effective? An analysis of integrated versus split treatment. *American Journal of Psychiatry, 156,* 324–326.

Dickersin, K. (1990). The existence of publication bias and risk factors for its occurrence. *JAMA, 263,* 1385–1389.

Doidge, N. (2007). *The brain that changes itself.* New York, NY: Viking.

Driessen, E., Hegelmaier, L. M., Abbass, A. A., Barber, J., Dekker, J., Van Henricus, L., . . . Cuijpers, P. (2015). The efficacy of short-term psychodynamic psychotherapy for depression: A meta-analysis update. *Clinical Psychology Review, 42*, 1–15.

Driessen, E., Hollon, S. D., Bockting, C. L. H., Cuijpers, P., & Turner, E. H. (2015, September 30). Does publication bias inflate the apparent efficacy of psychological treatment for major depressive disorder? A systematic review and meta-analysis of US National Institutes of Health-funded trials. *PLoS Medicine, 10*(9), e0137864.

Dunbar, R. I. M. (2014). The social brain: Psychological underpinnings and implications for the structure of organizations. *Current Directions in Psychological Science, 23*, 109–114.

Dutra, L., Stahopous, G., Basden, S. L., Leyr, T. M., Powers, M. B., & Otto, M. S. (2008). A meta-analytic review of psychosocial interventions for substance use disorders. *American Journal of Psychiatry, 165*, 179–187.

Eddington, A. (1928). *The nature of the physical world.* New York, NY: Macmillan.

Eisenberg, L. (1986). Mindlessness and brainlessness in psychiatry. *British Journal of Psychiatry, 148*, 497–508.

Eisenberg, L. (2000). Is psychiatry more mindful or brainier than it was a decade ago? *British Journal of Psychiatry, 176*, 1–5.

Elkin, I., Shea, T., Watkins, J. T., & Imber, S. D. (1989). National Institute of Mental Health Treatment of Depression Collaborative Research Program: General effectiveness of treatments. *Archives of General Psychiatry, 46*, 971–982.

Engel, G. L. (1980). The clinical application of the biopsychosocial model. *American Journal of Psychiatry, 137*, 535–544.

England, M. J., Butler, A. S., & Gonzalez, M. L. (Eds.). (2015). *Committee on Developing Evidence-Based Standards for Psychosocial Interventions for Mental Disorders.* Washington DC: National Academies Press.

Etain, B., Aas, M., Andreassen, O. A., Lorentzen, S., Dieset, I., Gard, S., . . . Henry, C. (2013). Childhood trauma is associated with severe clinical characteristics of bipolar disorders. *Journal of Clinical Psychiatry, 74*, 991–998.

Evidence-Based Medicine Working Group. (1992). Evidence-based medicine: A new approach to teaching the practice of medicine. *JAMA, 268*, 2420–2425.

Eysenck, H. (1952). The effects of psychotherapy: An evaluation. *Journal of Consulting Psychology, 16,* 319–324.

Fearon, P., Kirkbride, J. B., Morgan, C., Dazzan, R., & Murray, R. M. (2006). Incidence of schizophrenia and other psychoses in ethnic minority groups: Results from the MRC AESOP study. *Psychological Medicine, 36,* 1541–1550.

Fergusson, D. M., & Mullen, P. E. (1999). *Childhood sexual abuse: An evidence-based perspective.* Thousand Oaks, CA: Sage.

Fonagy, P. (2015). The effectiveness of psychodynamic psychotherapies: An update. *World Psychiatry, 14,* 137–150.

Fonagy, P., & Paris, J. (2008). Psychological treatments. In P. Tyrer & K Silk (Eds.), *Cambridge handbook of evidence-based psychiatric treatment.* Cambridge, England: Cambridge University Press.

Fournier, J. C., DeRubeis, R. J., Hollon, S. D., Dimidjian, S., Amsterdam, J. D., Shelton, R., & Fawcett, J. (2010). Antidepressant drug effects and depression severity: A patient-level meta-analysis. *JAMA, 303,* 47–53.

Frances, A. (2013). *Saving normal.* New York, NY: Morrow.

Frances, A. (2014). RDoC is necessary, but very oversold. *World Psychiatry, 13,* 47–48.

Frank, J. D., & Frank, J. B. (1991). *Persuasion and healing* (3rd ed.). Baltimore, MD: Johns Hopkins University Press.

Friston, K. J., Stephan, K. E., Montague, R., & Dolan, R. J. (2014). Computational psychiatry: The brain as a phantastic organ. *Lancet Psychiatry, 1,* 148–158.

Gabbard, G. O. (2009, September 3). Deconstructing the "Med Check." *Psychiatric Times.*

Gabbard, G. O., & Kay, J. (2001). The fate of integrated treatment: Whatever happened to the biopsychosocial psychiatrist? *American Journal of Psychiatry, 158,* 1956–1963.

Gabbard, G. O., Lazar, S. G., Hornberger, J., & Spiegel, D. (1997). The economic impact of psychotherapy: A review. *American Journal of Psychiatry, 154,* 147–155.

Gartlehner, G., Gaynes, B. N., Hansen, R. A., Thieda, P., DeVeaugh-Geiss, A., Krebs, E. E., . . . Lohr, K. L. (2008). Comparative benefits and harms of second-generation antidepressants: Background paper for the American College of Physicians. *Annals of Internal Medicine,149*, 734–750.

Gawande, A. (2014). *Being Mortal*. New York, Random House.

Gazzinaga, M., Ivry, R., & Mangun, G. R. (2002). *Cognitive neuroscience: The biology of the mind* (2nd ed.). New York, NY: Norton.

Geddes, J. R., Burgess, S., Hawton, K., Jamison, K., & Goodwin, G. M. (2004). Long-term lithium therapy for bipolar disorder: Systematic review and meta-analysis of randomized controlled trials. *American Journal of Psychiatry, 161*, 217–222.

Ghaemi, S. N. (2010). *The rise and fall of the biopsychosocial model: Reconciling art and science in psychiatry*. Baltimore, MD: Johns Hopkins University Press.

Glannon, W. (Ed.). (2015). *Free will and the brain: Neuroscientific, philosophical and legal perspectives*. Cambridge, England: Cambridge University Press.

Gold, I. (2009). Reduction in psychiatry. *Canadian Journal of Psychiatry, 54*, 506–512.

Goldberg, D., & Goodyer, I. (2005). *The origins and course of common mental disorders*. London, UK: Taylor & Francis.

Goldfried, M. R. (2016, February). On possible consequences of National Institute of Mental Health funding for psychotherapy research and training. *Professional Psychology: Research and Practice, 47*(1), 77–83.

Gould, S. D., & Lipkin, N. (1999). The doctor–patient relationship: Challenges, opportunities, and strategies. *Journal of General Internal Medicine, 14*(Suppl. 1), S26–S33.

Gyani, A., Shafran, R., Layard, R., & Clark, D. M. (2013). Enhancing recovery rates: Lessons from year one of IAPT. *Behaviour Research and Therapy, 51*, 597–606.

Hale, R. (1995). *The rise and crisis of psychoanalysis in the United States*. New York, NY: Oxford University Press.

Hamilton, M. (1960). A rating scale for depression. *Journal of Neurology, Neurosurgery and Psychiatry, 23*, 56–62.

Harding, C. M., Brooks, G. W., Ashikaga, T., Strauss, J. S., & Brier, A. (1987). Vermont Longitudinal Study of persons with severe mental illness. *American Journal of Psychiatry, 143*, 727–735.

Harris, G. (2011, March 6). Talk doesn't pay, so psychiatry turns instead to drug therapy. *The New York Times*.

Harris, J. R. (2009). *The nurture assumption: Why children turn out the way they do*, revised and updated. New York, NY: Simon & Schuster.

Healy, D. (1997). *The antidepressant era*. Cambridge, MA: Harvard University Press.

Healy, D. (2002). *The creation of psychopharmacology*. Cambridge, MA: Harvard University Press.

Hebb, D. O. (1949). *The organization of behavior*. New York, NY: Wiley.

Hickok, G. (2014). *The myth of mirror neurons: The real neuroscience of communication and cognition*. New York, NY: Norton.

Hollingshead, A., & Redlich, F. (1958). *Social class and mental illness*. New York, NY: Wiley.

Holmes, J. (2014). Psychodynamic psychiatry. In S. Bloch, S. Green, & J. Holmes (Eds.), *Psychiatry: Past, present and prospect* (pp. 420–432). New York, NY: Oxford University Press.

Horwitz, A. V., & Wakefield, J. C. (2007). *The loss of sadness: How psychiatry transformed normal sorrow into depressive disorder*. New York, NY: Oxford University Press.

Horwitz, A. V., & Wakefield, J. C. (2011). *All we have to fear: Psychiatry's transformation of natural anxieties into mental disorders*. New York, NY: Oxford University Press.

Horwitz, L. (1974). *Clinical prediction in psychotherapy*. New York, NY: Aronson.

Howard, K. I., Kopta, S. M., Krause, M. S., & Orlinsky, D. E. (1986). The dose–effect relationship to psychotherapy. *American Psychologist, 41*, 159–164.

Hyman, S. E. (2010). The diagnosis of mental disorders: The problem of reification. *Annual Review of Clinical Psychology, 6*, 155–179.

Hyman, S. E. (2012). Revolution stalled. *Science Translational Medicine, 4*(155), 155cm11.

Hyman, S. E. (2014a). Psychiatry and neuroscience. In S. Bloch, S. A. Green, & J. Holmes (Eds.), *Psychiatry: Past, present, and prospects* (pp. 4–21). New York, NY: Oxford University Press.

Hyman, S. E. (2014b). The unconscionable gap between what we know and what we do. *Science Translational Medicine, 4*, 1–5.

Insel, T., Cuthbert, B., Garvey, M., Heinssen, R., Pine, D. S., Quinn, K., & Wang, P. (2010). Research domain criteria: Toward a new classification framework for research on mental disorders. *American Journal of Psychiatry, 167*, 748–751.

Insel, T. R. (2015, February 10). Precision medicine for mental disorders. *Psychiatric Times.*

Insel, T. R., & Quirion, R. (2005). Psychiatry as a clinical neuroscience discipline. *JAMA, 294*, 2221–2224.

Insel, T. R., & Scolnick, E. M. (2006). Cure therapeutics and strategic prevention: Raising the bar for mental health research. *Molecular Psychiatry 11*, 11–17.

Institute of Medicine. (2015). *Psychosocial interventions for mental and substance use disorders: A framework for establishing evidence-based standards.* Washington, DC: National Academies Press.

Ioannidis, J. P. A. (2015). Research and theories on the etiology of mental diseases: Doomed to failure? *Psychological Inquiry, 26*, 239–243.

Jakobsen, J. L., Hansen, J. L., Simonsen, S., Simonsen, E., & Gluud, C. (2012). Effects of cognitive therapy versus interpersonal psychotherapy in patients with major depressive disorder: A systematic review of randomized clinical trials with meta-analyses and trial sequential analyses. *Psychological Medicine, 42*, 1343–1457.

Jacobson, N. S., Dobson, K. S., Truax, P. A., Addis, M. E., Koerner, K., Gollan, J. K., . . . Prince, S. E. (1996). A component analysis of cognitive–behavioral treatment for depression. *Journal of Consulting and Clinical Psychology, 64*, 295–304.

Jang, K. L. (2005). *The behavioral genetics of psychopathology: A clinical guide.* New York, NY: Routledge.

Kagan, J. (1997). *Galen's prophecy: Temperament in human nature.* Boulder, CO: Westview.

Kagan, J. (2006). *A young mind in a growing brain.* New York, NY: Psychology Press.

Kahneman, D. (2011). *Thinking fast and slow.* New York, NY: Macmillan.

Kandel, E. (1998). A new intellectual framework for psychiatry. *American Journal of Psychiatry, 155*, 457–469.

Kane, J. M., Robinson, D. G., & Schooler, D. (2016). Comprehensive versus usual community care for first episode psychosis: Two-year outcomes from the NIMH RAISE early treatment program. *American Journal of Psychiatry, 173*, 362–372.

Kantor, E. D., Rehm, C. D., Haas, J. S., Chan, A. T., & Giovannucci, E. L. (2015). Trends in prescription drug use among adults in the United States from 1999–2012. *JAMA, 314*, 1818–1830.

Kates, N., Craven, M., Bishop, J., Clinton, T., Kraftcheck, D., & LeClair, K. (2006). Shared mental health care in Canada. *Canadian Journal of Psychiatry, 56*(Suppl. 1), 21–67.

Kauffman, S. (1993). *The origins of order: Self-organization and selection in evolution.* New York, NY: Oxford University Press.

Kauffman, S. (1995). *At home in the universe: The search for the laws of self-organization and complexity.* New York, NY: Oxford University Press.

Kazdin, A. E. (2008). Evidence-based treatment and practice: New opportunities to bridge clinical research and practice, enhance the knowledge base, and improve patient care. *American Psychologist, 63*, 146–149.

Keller, M. B., Ryan, N. D., Strober, M., Klein, R. G., Kutcher, S. P., & Birmaher, B. (2001). Efficacy of Paroxetine in the Treatment of Adolescent Major Depression: A Randomized, Controlled Trial. *Journal of the American Academy of Child and Adolescent Psychiatry, 40*, 762–772.

Kendler, K. S., & Prescott, C. A. (2006). *Genes, environment, and psychopathology: Understanding the causes of psychiatric and substance use disorders.* New York, NY: Guilford.

Kennedy, S. H., Lam, R. W., Patten, S. B., & Ravindran, A. V. (2009). Canadian Network for Mood and Anxiety Treatments (CANMAT) clinical guidelines for the management of major depressive disorder in adults. *Journal of Affective Disorders, 117*, S1–S2.

Kessler, R. C., Berglundd, P., Demier, O., Jin, R., Merikangas, K. R., & Walters, E. E. (2005). Lifetime prevalence and age-of-onset distributions of DSM-IV disorders in the National Comorbidity Survey Replication. *Archives of General Psychiatry, 62*, 593–602.

Kessler, R. C., Davis, C. G., & Kendler, K. S. (1997). Childhood adversity and adult psychiatric disorder in the US National Comorbidity Survey. *Psychological Medicine, 27*, 1101–1119.

Khan, A., & Brown, W. A. (2015). Antidepressants versus placebo in major depression: An overview. *World Psychiatry, 14,* 294–300.

Kingsbury, S. J., Yi, S., & Simpson, G. M. (2001). Psychopharmacology: Rational and irrational polypharmacy. *Psychiatric Services, 52,* 1033–1036.

Kirmayer, L. J. (2015). Re-visioning psychiatry: Toward an ecology of mind in health and illness. In L. J. Kirmayer, R. Lemelson, & C. A. Cummings (Eds.), *Re-visioning psychiatry: Cultural phenomenology, critical neuroscience and global mental health.* New York, NY: Cambridge University Press.

Kirmayer, L. J., & Crafa, D. (2014). What kind of science for psychiatry? *Frontiers in Human Neuroscience, 8,* 435–440.

Kirmayer, L. J., & Gold, I. (2012). Critical neuroscience and the limits of reductionism. In S. Choudury & J Slaby (Eds.), *Critical neuroscience: A handbook of the social and cultural contexts of neuroscience* (pp. 307–330). New York, NY: Wiley-Blackwell.

Kirsch, I. (2014). Antidepressants and the placebo effect. *Zeitschrift fur Psychologie, 222,* 128–134.

Kirsch, I., Deacon, B. J., Huedo-Medina, T. B., Scoboria, A., Moore, T. J., & Johnson, B. T. (2008). Initial severity and antidepressant benefits: a meta-analysis of data submitted to the Food and Drug Administration. *PLoS Medicine, 5,* e45.

Kleinman, A. (1988). *Rethinking psychiatry: From cultural category to personal experience.* New York, NY: Free Press.

Klerman, G. L. (1990). The psychiatric patient's right to effective treatment: Implications of *Osheroff v. Chestnut Lodge. American Journal of Psychiatry, 147,* 409–418.

Knekt, P., Heinonen, E., Harkapaa, K., Virtala, E., Rissannen, J., & Lindfors, O. (2015). Randomized trial on the effectiveness of short- and long-term psychotherapy on psychosocial functioning and quality of life during a 5-year follow-up. *Psychiatry Research, 229,* 381–388.

Komossa, K., Depping, A. M., Gaudchau, A., Kissling, W., & Leucht, S. (2010, December 8). Second-generation antipsychotics for major depressive disorder and dysthymia. *Cochrane Database of Systematic Reviews* (12), CD008121.

Kraepelin, E: Dementia Praecox and Paraphrenia (1919) Edinburgh, E. & S. Livingstone.

Lam, R., Kennedy, S. J., Grigoriadis, S., McIntyre, R. S., Milev, R., Ramasubbu, R., ... Ravindran, A. V. (2009). Canadian Network for Mood and Anxiety Treatments (CANMAT) clinical guidelines for the management of major depressive disorder in adults: III. Pharmacotherapy. *Journal of Affective Disorders Supplement*, S26–S43.

Lambert, M. (Ed.). (2013). *Bergin and Garfield's handbook of psychotherapy and behavior change* (6th ed.). New York, NY: Wiley.

Laporte, L., Paris, J., Russell, J., & Guttman, H. (2011). Psychopathology, trauma, and personality traits in patients with borderline personality disorder and their sisters. *Journal of Personality Disorders, 25*, 448, 462.

Lashley, K. (1950). In search of the engram. *Society of Experimental Biology Symposium, 4*, 454–482.

Lazar, S. G. (Ed.). (2010). *Psychotherapy is worth it: A comprehensive review of its cost-effectiveness*. Washington, DC: American Psychiatric Publishing.

Lehmann, H. E. (1986). The future of psychiatry: Progress—mutation—or self destruct? *Canadian Journal of Psychiatry, 31*, 362–367.

Leichsenring, F., & Rabung, S. (2008). Effectiveness of long-term psychodynamic psychotherapy: A meta-analysis. *JAMA, 300*, 1551–1565.

Leichsenring, F., & Rabung, S. (2011). Long-term psychodynamic psychotherapy in complex mental disorders: Update of a meta-analysis. *British Journal of Psychiatry, 199*, 15–22.

Leichsenring, F., & Rabung, S. (2011). Long-term psychodynamic psychotherapy in complex mental disorders: update of a meta-analysis. *The British Journal of Psychiatry, 199*, 15–22.

Leichsenring, F., Rabung, S., & Leibing, E. (2004). The efficacy of short-term psychodynamic psychotherapy in specific psychiatric disorders: A meta-analysis. *Archives of General Psychiatry, 61*, 1208–1216.

LeNoury, J., Nardo, J. M., Healy, D., Jureidini, J., Raven, M., Tufananaru, T., & Abi-Jaoude, E. (2015). Restoring Study 329: Efficacy and harms of paroxetine and imipramine in treatment of major depression in adolescence. *BMJ, 351*, h4320.

Leucht, S., Hierl, S., Kissling, W., Dold, M., & Davis, J. M. (2012). Putting the efficacy of psychiatric and general medicine medication into perspective: Review of meta-analyses. *British Journal of Psychiatry, 200,* 97–106.

Lewis, S., & Lieberman, J. A. (2008). CATIE and CUtLASS: Can we handle the truth? *British Journal of Psychiatry, 192,* 161–163.

Libet, B., Gleason, C. A., Wright, E. W., & Pearl, D. K. (1983). Time of conscious intention to act in relation to onset of cerebral activity (readiness-potential)—The unconscious initiation of a freely voluntary act. *Brain, 106,* 623–642.

Lieberman, J. A., Stroup, T. S., McEvoy, J. P., Swartz, M. S., Rosenheck, R. A., Perkins, D. O., and the Clinical Antipsychotic Trials of Intervention Effectiveness (CATIE) Investigators. (2005). Effectiveness of antipsychotic drugs in patients with chronic schizophrenia. *New England Journal of Medicine, 353,* 1209–1223.

Lilienfeld, S. O. (2014). The Research Domain Criteria (RDoC): An analysis of methodological and conceptual challenges. *Behaviour Research and Therapy, 62,* 129–139.

Linden, D. E. (2006). How psychotherapy changes the brain—The contribution of functional neuroimaging. *Molecular Psychiatry, 11,* 528–538.

Linehan, M. M., Korslund, K. E., Harned, M. S., Gallop, R. J., Lungu, A., Neacsiu, A. D., . . . Murray-Gregory, A. M. (2015). Dialectical behavior therapy for high suicide risk in individuals with borderline personality disorder: A randomized clinical trial and component analysis. *JAMA Psychiatry, 72,* 475–482.

Logothetis, N. K. (2008). What we can do and what we cannot do with fMRI. *Nature, 453,* 869–878.

Luborsky, L., Singer, B., & Luborsky, L. (1975). Comparative studies of psychotherapies: Is it true that "everyone has won and all must have prizes"? *Archives of General Psychiatry, 32,* 995–1008.

Luhrmann, T. (2000). *Of two minds.* New York, NY: Norton.

Lundgren, M., Charpentier, E., & Fineran, P. C. (2015). *CRISPR: Methods and protocols.* New York, NY: Springer.

Lyons, Z. (2013). Attitudes of medical students toward psychiatry and psychiatry as a career: A systematic review. *Academic Psychiatry, 37,* 150–157.

MacGillivray, S., Arroll, B., Hatcher, S., & Ogston, S. (2003). Efficacy and tolerability of selective serotonin reuptake inhibitors compared with tricyclic antidepressants in depression treated in primary care: Systematic review and meta-analysis. *BMJ, 326,* 1014–1017.

MacKenzie, K. R. (1996). The time-limited psychotherapies: An overview. *American Psychiatric Press Review of Psychiatry, 15*, 11–21.

Marcus, S. C., & Olfson, M. (2010). National trends in the treatment for depression from 1998 to 2007. *Archives of General Psychiatry, 67*, 1265–1273.

Markowitz, J. C. (2016, October 14). There's such a thing as too much neuroscience. *The New York Times*.

Markowitz, J. C., & Milrod, B. (2011). The importance of responding to negative affect in psychotherapies. *American Journal of Psychiatry, 168*, 124–128.

Markowitz, J. C., & Weissman, M. M. (2015). Interpersonal psychotherapy: Past, present and future. *Clinical Psychology & Psychotherapy, 19*, 99–105.

McCallum, M., & Piper, W. E. (Eds.). (1997). *Psychological mindedness: A contemporary understanding*. Munich, Germany: Erlbaum.

McClellan, J. M., Susser, E., & King, M. C. (2007). Schizophrenia: A common disease caused by multiple rare alleles. *British Journal of Psychiatry, 190*, 194–199.

McGowan, P. O., & Roth, T. L. (2015). Epigenetic pathways through which experiences become linked with biology. *Development and Psychopathology, 27*, 637–648.

McHugh, P. R., & Slavney, P. R. (1998). *The perspectives of psychiatry* (2nd ed.). Baltimore, MD: Johns Hopkins University Press.

McHugh, R. K., Whitton, S. W., Peckham, A. D., Welge, J. A., & Ottos, M. W. (2013). Patient preference for psychological vs. pharmacological treatment of psychiatric disorders: A meta-analytic review. *Journal of Clinical Psychiatry, 74*, 595–602.

McKenzie, K., & Shah, J. (2015). Understanding the social etiology of psychosis. In L. J. Kirmayer, R. Lemelson, & C. A. Cummings (Eds.), *Re-visioning psychiatry: Cultural phenomenology, critical neuroscience, and global mental health* (pp. 317–342). New York, NY: Cambridge University Press.

McLaren, N. (1998). A critical review of the biopsychosocial model. *Australasian Psychiatry, 32*, 86–92.

McMain, S. F., Links, P. S., Gnam, W. H., Guimond, T., Cardish, R. J., Korman, L., & Streiner, D. L. (2009). A randomized trial of dialectical behavior therapy versus general psychiatric management for borderline personality disorder. *American Journal of Psychiatry, 166*, 1365–1374.

McNally, R. J. (2003). *Remembering trauma.* Cambridge, MA: Belknap/Harvard University Press.

Mead, N., Lester, H., Chew-Graham, C., & Gask, L. (2010). Effects of befriending on depressive symptoms and distress: Systematic review and meta-analysis. *British Journal of Psychiatry, 196*, 96–101.

Meaney, M. J., & Szyf, M. (2005). Environmental programming of stress responses through DNA methylation: Life at the interface between a dynamic environment and a fixed genome. *Dialogues in Clinical Neuroscience, 7*, 103–123.

Meloni, M., & Testa, G. (2014). Scrutinizing the epigenetics revolution. *BioSocieties, 9*, 431–456.

Men, W., Falk, D., Sun, T., Chen, W., Li, J., Yin, D. . . . Fan, M. (2014). The corpus callosum of Albert Einstein's brain: Another clue to his high intelligence? *Brain, 137*(Pt. 4), e268.

Mental Health Commission of Canada. (2012). *Changing directions, changing lives.* Retrieved from http://strategy.mentalhealthcommission.ca

Miller, W. R., & Rollnick, S. (2002). *Motivational interviewing* (2nd ed.). New York, NY: Guilford.

Mojtabai, R., & Olfson, M. (2008). National trends in psychotherapy by office-based psychiatrists. *Archives of General Psychiatry, 65*, 962–970.

Mojtabai, R., & Olfson, M. (2010). National trends in psychotropic medication polypharmacy in office-based psychiatry. *Archives of General Psychiatry, 67*, 26–36.

Moncrieff, J. (2009). A critique of the dopamine hypothesis of schizophrenia and psychosis. *Harvard Review of Psychiatry, 17*, 214–225.

Moncrieff, J., Wessely, S., & Hardy, R. (2004). Active placebos versus antidepressants for depression. *Cochrane Database of Systematic Reviews* (1), CD003012.

Murphy, R., Straebler, S., Cooper, Z., & Fairburn, C. G. (2010). Cognitive behavioral therapy for eating disorders. *Psychiatric Clinics of North America, 33*, 611–627.

National Institute for Care Excellence. (2009). *Depression in adults: The treatment and management of depression in adults.* Retrieved from https://www.nice.org.uk/guidance/cg90

Nelson, J. C., & Papakostas, G. I. (2009). Atypical antipsychotic augmentation in major depressive disorder: A meta-analysis of placebo-controlled randomized trials. *American Journal of Psychiatry, 166,* 980–991.

Nesse, R. M. (2005). Evolutionary explanations for mood and mood disorders. In D. Stein, D. J. Kupfer, & A. Schatzberg (Eds.), *The American Psychiatric Publishing Textbook of Mood Disorders* (pp. 159–175). Washington, DC: American Psychiatric Publishing.

Newton-Howes, G., Tyrer, P., & Johnson, T. (2006). Personality disorder and the outcome of depression: Meta-analysis of published studies. *British Journal of Psychiatry, 188,* 13–20.

Norcross, J. C., & Goldfried, M. R. (2005). *Handbook of psychotherapy integration* (2nd ed.). New York, NY: Oxford University Press.

O'Donnell, M. (1997). *A skeptic's medical dictionary.* London, UK: BMJ Publishing Group.

Olfson, M., Blanco, C., Liu, M. S., Wang, S., & Correll, C. U. (2012). National trends in the office-based treatment of children, adolescents, and adults with antipsychotics. *Archives of General Psychiatry, 69,* 1247–1256.

Olfson, M., & Marcus, S. C. (2010). National trends in outpatient psychotherapy. *American Journal of Psychiatry, 167,* 1456–1463.

Orlinsky, D. E., Grawe, K., & Parks, B. K. (1994). Process and outcome in psychotherapy—Noch einmal. In A. E. Bergin & S. L. Garfield (Eds.), *Handbook of psychotherapy and behavior change* (4th ed., pp. 270–379). New York, NY: Wiley.

Ost, L. G. (2008). Efficacy of the third wave of behavioral therapies: A systematic review and meta-analysis. *Behaviour Research and Therapy, 46,* 296–321.

Panksepp, J., & Harro, J. (2004). Future of neuropeptides in biological psychiatry and emotional psychopharmacology: Goals and strategies. In J. Panksepp (Ed.), *Textbook of biological psychiatry* (pp. 627–659). New York, NY: Wiley.

Papakostas, G. I., & Fava, M. (2010). *Pharmacotherapy for depression and treatment-resistant depression.* Hackensack, NJ: World Scientific.

Paris, J. (1999). *Nature and nurture in psychiatry.* Washington, DC: American Psychiatric Publishing.

Paris, J. (2000). *Myths of childhood.* Philadelphia, PA: Brunner/Mazel.

Paris, J. (2005). *The fall of an icon: Psychoanalysis and academic psychiatry.* Toronto, Ontario, Canada: University of Toronto Press.

Paris, J. (2008). *Prescriptions for the mind; A critical view of contemporary psychiatry.* New York, NY: Oxford University Press.

Paris, J. (2010a). *The use and misuse of psychiatric drugs: An evidence-based guide.* London, UK: Wiley.

Paris, J. (2010b). Effectiveness of differing psychotherapy approaches in the treatment of borderline personality disorder. *Current Psychiatry Reports, 12,* 56–60.

Paris, J. (2013). Stepped care for patients with borderline personality disorder. *Psychiatric Services, 64,* 1035–1037.

Paris, J. (2015a). *The intelligent clinician's guide to DSM-5* (2nd ed.). New York, NY: Oxford University Press.

Paris, J. (2015b). *Overdiagnosis in psychiatry.* New York, NY: Oxford University Press.

Paris, J. (2015c). Applying the principles of psychotherapy integration to the treatment of borderline personality disorder. *Journal of Psychotherapy Integration, 25,* 13–19.

Paris, J., Bhat, V., & Thombs, B. (2015). Is adult ADHD being overdiagnosed? *Canadian Journal of Psychiatry, 60,* 324–328.

Paris, J., Goldbloom, D. & Kurdyak, P. (2015). Moving out of the office: Problems in access to psychiatry. *Canadian Journal of Psychiatry, 60,* 403–406.

Paris, J., & Kirmayer, L. J. (2016). The research domain criteria—A bridge too far? *Journal of Nervous and Mental Diseases, 204*(1), 26–32.

Parker, G., & Manicavasagar, V. (2005). *Modelling and managing the depressive disorders: A clinical guide.* Cambridge, England: Cambridge University Press.

Parnas, J. (2014). Psychiatry without the psyche. *World Psychiatry, 13,* 46–47.

Pascual-Leone, A., Amedi, A., Fregni, F., & Merabet, L. B. (2005). The plastic human brain cortex. *Annual Review of Neuroscience, 28*, 377–401.

Peterson, B. S. (2015). Research Domain Criteria (RDoC): A new psychiatric nosology whose time has not yet come. *Journal of Child Psychology and Psychiatry, 56*, 719–722.

Pies, R. (2005). Why psychiatry and neurology cannot simply merge. *Journal of Neuropsychiatry and Clinical Neurosciences, 17*, 304–309.

Pigott, H. E., Leventhal, A. M., Alter, G. S., & Boren, J. J. (2010). Efficacy and effectiveness of antidepressants: Current status of research. *Psychotherapy and Psychosomatics, 79*, 267–279.

Pilgrim, D. (2002). The biopsychosocial model in Anglo-American psychiatry: Past, present and future. *Journal of Mental Health, 11*(6), 585–594.

Pincus, H. A., Tanielian, T. L., Marcus, S. C., Olfson, M., Zarin, D. A., Thompson, J., & Magno Zito, J. (1998). Prescribing trends in psychotropic medications: Primary care, psychiatry, and other medical specialties. *JAMA, 279*, 526–531.

Pinker, S. (1997). *How the mind works.* New York, NY: Norton.

Pinker, S. (2002). *The blank slate.* New York, NY: Penguin.

Plakun, E. (2015). Psychotherapy and psychosocial treatment: Recent advances and future directions. *Psychiatric Clinics of North America, 38*, 405–418.

Plomin, R., DeFries, J. C., Knopik, V. S., & Neiderhiser, J. M. (2013). *Behavioral genetics* (6th ed.). London, UK: Palgrave Macmillan.

Poldrack, R. A. (2006). Can cognitive processes be inferred from neuroimaging data? *Trends in Cognitive Science, 10*, 59–63.

Popper, K. (1968). *Conjectures and refutations.* New York, NY: Harper Torch.

Pratt, L. A., Brody, D. J., & Gu, Q. (2011). *Antidepressant use in persons aged 12 and over: United States, 2005–2008* (NCHS data brief no 76). Hyattsville, MD: National Center for Health Statistics.

Price, B. H., Adams, R. D., & Coyle, J. T. (2000). Neurology and psychiatry: Closing the great divide. *Neurology, 54*, 8–14.

Prochaska, J. O., Norcross, J. C., & DiClemente, C. C. (1994). *Changing for good.* New York, NY: Morrow.

Propst, A., Paris, J., & Rosberger, Z. (1994). Do therapist experience, diagnosis, and functional level predict outcome in short-term psychotherapy? *Canadian Journal of Psychiatry, 39,* 178–183.

Raz, A. (2012). From neuroimaging to tea leaves in the bottom of a cup. In S. Choudhury & J. Slaby (Eds.), *Critical neuroscience* (pp. 265–270). New York, NY: Wiley-Blackwell.

Regier, D. A., Narrow, W. E., Clarke, D. E., Kraekere, H. C., Kuramoto, J., Kuhl, E. A., & Kupfer, D. J. (2013). DSM-5 field trials in the United States and Canada, Part II: Test–retest reliability of selected categorical diagnoses. *American Journal of Psychiatry, 170,* 59–70.

Regier, D. A., Narrow, W., Rae, D., Manderscheid, R., Locke, B., & Goodwin, F. K. (1993). The de Facto US mental and addictive disorders system: Epidemiologic catchment area prospective 1-year prevalence rates of disorders and services. *Archives of General Psychiatry, 50,* 85–94.

Richards, D. A. (2012). Stepped care: A method to deliver increased access to psychological therapies. *Canadian Journal of Psychiatry, 57,* 210–215.

Rogers, C. (1951). *Client-centered therapy: Its current practice, implications and theory.* London, UK: Constable.

Rosenzweig, S. (1936). Some implicit common factors in diverse methods of psychotherapy: "At last the Dodo said, 'Everybody has won and all must have prizes.'" *American Journal of Orthopsychiatry, 6,* 412–415.

Rossler, W. (2006). Psychiatric rehabilitation today: An overview. *World Psychiatry, 5,* 151–157.

Roth, A., & Fonagy, P. (2005). *What works for whom? A critical review of psychotherapy research* (2nd ed.). New York, NY: Guilford.

Ruge, D., Liou, L.-M., & Hoad, D. (2012). Improving the potential of neuroplasticity. *Journal of Neuroscience, 32,* 5705–5706.

Rush, A. J. (2007). STAR*D: What have we learned? *American Journal of Psychiatry, 164,* 201–204.

Rush, B., McPherson-Does, C., Behroozm, R. C., & Cudmore, A. (2013). Exploring core competencies for mental health and addictions work within a Family Health Team setting. *Mental Health in Family Medicine, 10,* 89–100.

Rutter, M. (2000). Psychosocial influences: Critiques, findings, and research needs. *Development and Psychopathology, 12,* 375–405.

Rutter, M. (2006). *Genes and behavior: Nature–nurture interplay explained.* London, UK: Blackwell.

Rutter, M. (2012). Resilience as a dynamic concept. *Development and Psychopathology, 24,* 335–344.

Rutter, M., & Rutter, M. (1993). *Developing Minds: Challenge and Continuity Across the Life Span.* New York, Basic.

Rutter, M., Kumsta, R., Schlotz, W., & Sonuga-Barke, E. (2012). Longitudinal studies using a "natural experiment" design: The case of adoptees from Romanian institutions. *Journal of the American Academy of Child & Adolescent Psychiatry, 51,* 762–770.

Sackett, D. L., Richardson, W. S., Rosenberg, W., & Haynes, R. B. (1997). *Evidence-based medicine.* Edinburgh, UK: Churchill Livingstone.

Sapolsky, R. (2003). Gene therapy in psychiatry. *American Journal of Psychiatry, 160,* 208–220.

Sareen, J., Cox, B., Afifi, T., Yu, B., & Stein, M. (2005). Mental health service use in a nationally representative Canadian survey. *Canadian Journal of Psychiatry, 50,* 753–761.

Satel, S., & Lilienfeld, S. (2013). *Brainwashed: The seductive appeal of mindless neuroscience.* New York, NY: Basic Books.

Schizophrenia Working Group of the Psychiatric Genetics Consortium. (2014). Biological insights from 108 schizophrenia-associated genetic loci. *Nature, 511,* 421–427.

Schmidt, N. B., Korte, K. J., Norr, A. M., Keough, M. E., & Timpano, K. R. (2014). Panic disorder and agoraphobia. In P. Emmelkamp & T. Ehring (Eds.), *The Wiley handbook of anxiety disorders* (pp. 321–356). New York, NY: Wiley.

Schofield, P. (1964). *Psychotherapy: The purchase of friendship.* New York, NY: Prentice Hall.

Schwartz, S. J., Lilienfeld, S. O., Meca, A., & Sauvigne, K. C. (2016). The role of neuroscience within psychology: A call for inclusiveness over exclusiveness. *American Psychologist, 71*, 52–70.

Scull, A. Madness in Civilization (2015). A Cultural History of Insanity, from the Bible to Freud, from the Madhouse to Modern Medicine. Princeton NJ, Princeton Univ Press.

Segal, Z., Williams, M. G., & Teasdale, J. D. (Eds.). (2013). *Mindfulness based cognitive therapy for depression* (2nd ed.). New York, NY: Guilford.

Shorter, E. (1997). *A history of psychiatry; From the era of the asylum to the age of Prozac.* New York, NY: Wiley.

Smith, M. L., Glass, G. V., & Miller, T. (1980). *The benefits of psychotherapy.* Baltimore, MD: Johns Hopkins University Press.

Spielmans, G. I., Berman, M. I., Linardatos, E., Rosenlicht, N. Z., Perry, A., & Tsai, A. C. (2013). Adjunctive atypical antipsychotic treatment for major depressive disorder: A meta-analysis of depression, quality of life, and safety outcomes. *PLOS Medicine, 10*(3), e1001403.

Stevens, E. S., Jendrusina, A. A., Sarapas, C., & Behar, E. (2014). Generalized anxiety disorder. In P. Emmelkamp & T. Ehring (Eds.), *The Wiley handbook of anxiety disorders* (pp. 378–423). New York, NY: Wiley.

Stiles, W. B., Barkham, M., & Wheeler, S. (2015). Duration of psychological therapy: Relation to recovery and improvement rates in UK routine practice. *British Journal of Psychiatry, 207*, 115–122.

Strupp, H. H., & Hadley, S. W. (1979). Specific vs. non-specific factors in psychotherapy. *Archives General Psychiatry, 36*, 1125–1136.

Tarrier, N. (2005). Cognitive behavior therapy for schizophrenia— A review of development, evidence and implementation. *Psychotherapy & Psychosomatics, 74*, 136–144.

Taylor, M. (2013). *Hippocrates Cried.* New York, NY: Oxford University Press.

Thornton, L. M., Mazzeo, S. E., & Bulik, C. M. (2010). The Heritability of Eating Disorders: Methods and Current Findings. *Current Topics in Behavioral Neurosciences, 6*, 141–156.

Torgersen, S., Lygren, S., Oien, P. A., Skre, I., Onstad, S., & Edvardsen, J. (2000). A twin study of personality disorders. *Comprehensive Psychiatry, 41*, 416–425.

True, W. R., Rice, J., Eisen, S. A., Heath, A. C., Goldberg, J., Lyons, M. J., & Nowak, J. (1993). A twin study of genetic and environmental contributions to liability for post-traumatic stress symptoms. *Archives of General Psychiatry, 50,* 257–264.

van Essen, D. C., & Barch, D. M. (2015). The human connectome in health and psychopathology. *World Psychiatry, 14,* 154–157.

van Os, J., Lataster, T., Delespaul, P., Wichers, M., & Myin-Germeys, I. (2014). Evidence that a psychopathology interactome has diagnostic value, predicting clinical needs: An experience sampling study. *Neurodynamics, 4,* 575–581.

Wahlbeck, K., Cheine, M. V., & Essali, A. (2000). Clozapine versus typical neuroleptic medication for schizophrenia. *Cochrane Database of Systematic Reviews* (2), CD000059.

Wampold, B. E. (2015). *The great psychotherapy debate: Models, methods, and findings,* 2nd edition. Mahwah, NJ: Erlbaum.

Weissman, M., Verdekui, H. M., & Gameroff, M. J. (2006). National survey of psychotherapy training in psychiatry, psychology, and social work. *Archives of General Psychiatry, 63,* 925–934.

Westen, D., & Morrison, K. (2001). A multidimensional meta-analysis of treatments for depression, panic, and generalized anxiety disorder: An empirical examination of the status of empirically supported therapies. *J Consulting & Clinical Psychology, 69,* 875–899.

Wilson, E. O. (1994). *Naturalist.* Washington, DC: Island Press.

Wilson, G. T., Grilo, C. M., & Vitousek, K. M. (2007). Psychological treatment of eating disorders. *American Psychologist, 62,* 199–216.

Wilson, G. T., Vitousek, K. M., & Loeb, K. L. (2000). Stepped care treatment for eating disorders. *Journal of Consulting and Clinical Psychology, 68,* 564–572.

Woolfolk, R. L. (2015). *The value of psychotherapy: The talking cure in an age of clinical science.* New York, NY: Guilford.

Wright, J. H., Sudak, D. M., Turkington, D., & Thase, M. (Eds.). (2010). *High-yield cognitive–behavior therapy for brief sessions.* Washington, DC: American Psychiatric Publishing.

Wunderink, L., Neboer, R. M., Wierma, D., Sytema, C., & Nienhuis, F. J. (2013). Recovery in remitted first-episode psychosis at 7 years of follow-up of an early dose reduction/discontinuation or maintenance treatment strategy: Long-term follow-up of a 2-year randomized clinical trial. *JAMA Psychiatry, 70*, 913–920.

Yanai, I., & Lercher, M. (2016). *The society of genes.* Cambridge, MA: Harvard University Press.

Yudofsky, S., & Hales, R. (2002). Neuropsychiatry and the future of psychiatry and neurology. *American Journal of Psychiatry, 159,* 1261–1264.

Zachar, P. (2000). *Biological psychiatry: A philosophical analysis.* Philadelphia, PA: Benjamins.

Zimmerman, M., Chelminski, I., & Young, D. (2008). The frequency of personality disorders in psychiatric patients. *Psychiatric Clinics of North America, 31*, 405–420.

Zimmerman, M., Mattia, J., & Posternak, M. A. (2002). Are subjects in pharmacological treatment trials of depression representative of patients in routine clinical practice? *American Journal of Psychiatry, 159,* 469–473.

INDEX